Milestones in Drug Therapy

For further volumes:
http://www.springer.com/series/4991

Maria Sibilia • Christoph C. Zielinski •
Rupert Bartsch • Thomas W. Grunt
Editors

Drugs for HER-2-positive Breast Cancer

Springer

Volume Editors
Prof. Dr. Maria Sibilia
Comprehensive Cancer Center
Institute of Cancer Research
Department of Medicine I
Medical University of Vienna
Borschkegasse 8a
1090 Vienna
Austria
Maria.Sibilia@meduniwien.ac.at

Prof. Dr. Christoph C. Zielinski
Comprehensive Cancer Center
Department of Medicine I
Medical University of Vienna
General Hospital
Waehringer Guertel 18-20
1090 Vienna
Austria
christoph.zielinski@meduniwien.ac.at

Dr. Rupert Bartsch
Comprehensive Cancer Center
Department of Medicine I
Clinical Division of Oncology
Medical University of Vienna
Waehringer Guertel 18-20
1090 Vienna
Austria
rupert.bartsch@meduniwien.ac.at

Assoc. Prof. Dr. Thomas W. Grunt, PH.D.
Comprehensive Cancer Center
Department of Medicine I
Clinical Division of Oncology
Medical University of Vienna
Waehringer Guertel 18-20
1090 Vienna
Austria
thomas.grunt@meduniwien.ac.at

Series Editors
Prof. Dr. Michael J. Parnham
Director of Science & Technology
MediMlijeko d.o.o.
Pozarinje 7
HR-10000 Zagreb
Croatia

Prof. Dr. Jacques Bruinvels
Sweelincklaan 75
NL-3723 JC Bilthoven
The Netherlands

ISBN 978-3-0348-0318-2 ISBN 978-3-0346-0094-1 (eBook)
DOI 10.1007/978-3-0346-0094-1

Cover design: deblik, Berlin

Printed on acid-free paper

Springer Basel AG is part of Springer Science + Business Media (www.springer.com)

Preface

Drugs for HER-2-positive Breast Cancer: A Major Approval for Translational Cancer Research

Research over the last 2–3 decades in the fields of cell and molecular biology as well as biomedicine has tremendously improved our understanding of the mechanisms of malignant transformation and progression. A lot of knowledge gained from these findings could already be transferred to clinical application and has led to a number of major advances in the early diagnosis and treatment of cancer. This applies especially to breast cancer. Development of molecular-targeted drugs nowadays is characterized by several key features. In the first step, promising molecular targets have to be identified. The ideal cancer drug target – albeit not often found – should represent a molecule that is absolutely required for the proliferation and survival of the transformed cell. In other words, it should be a molecule to which the tumour cell is "addicted" (the "Achilles heel"). Consequently, the choice of drug targets is based on and driven by a profound knowledge about the cellular and molecular biology of the crucial regulatory processes that are significantly aberrant in malignant cells. In the second step, promising chemical lead structures are identified or a panel of antibodies is produced. Therefore, whereas classical cytotoxic drugs were previously identified by more or less random screening of large libraries of (natural and synthetic) compounds, novel molecular-targeted drugs are usually identified by a more rational approach that takes into account several aspects such as the physical–chemical properties of the aimed target domain and the therapeutic compound. These agents are then screened for optimal therapeutic indexes (maximal treatment effects with concurrent minimal side effects).

Tamoxifen was the first molecular-targeted drug ever in use in clinical oncology. It has been and is still being used for the management of oestrogen receptor-positive breast tumours. This drug – originally developed as an oral contraceptive – was not successful for that indication. However, "by chance" it was found that tamoxifen potently blocks the growth of oestrogen receptor-positive breast cancer cells [1]. In contrast to tamoxifen, development of the anti-ErbB2 antibody trastuzumab against ErbB2-positive metastatic breast cancer was "hypothesis-driven" according to the above-mentioned criteria. Thus, trastuzumab became the first clinically available oncogene-targeted therapeutic agent for the treatment of solid tumours (see chapter by Bartsch and Steger). The first kinase inhibitor for application against malignant diseases was imatinib. It inhibits the ABL kinase, which is rearranged and hyperactive in chronic myelogenous leukaemia. Notably, recent encouraging data indicate that the reversible dual-specific EGFR/ErbB2 kinase inhibitor lapatinib is still effective in ErbB2-positive breast cancer patients who have already developed resistance to trastuzumab. In conclusion, breast cancer belongs to that type of solid tumours, in which molecular-targeted therapies were most efficient and yielded most clinical benefits so far (e.g. tamoxifen, trastuzumab, lapatinib). Unfortunately, however, despite these improvements, breast cancer is still a major life-threatening disease for women in industrialized as well as developing countries, and there are several significant detriments when using ErbB-targeted therapies against mammary cancer. First, only a proportion of ErbB2-positive breast cancers are actually sensitive to trastuzumab (a priori, primary resistance). Moreover, almost all ErbB2-positive, trastuzumab-sensitive breast cancers become resistant within 1 year of trastuzumab treatment (acquired, secondary resistance) (see chapters by Morgillo et al., Bianchi and Gianni, von Minckwitz and Pirvulescu). In recent years, it has become increasingly evident that signalling pathways are by no means linear cascades of signal processing; they rather represent intensely interwoven regulatory networks that communicate with each other via several relay proteins that function as signalling hubs (see chapter by Köstler and Yarden). Thus, even if a highly specific drug such as trastuzumab potently silences its intended target ErbB2, the cell still might be capable of avoiding the growth-inhibitory pressure by rerouting the signal to other growth-promoting cascades leading to resistance after a certain treatment period. Therefore, targeted cancer treatment should seek to specifically neutralise the hub proteins, which control a number of signal pathways that are crucial for cancer cell growth and survival (the "Achilles heel" of cancer). Another possibility is to use kinase inhibitors with broader specificity in order to neutralize more than one signalling protein. Novel treatment strategies usually apply more than one targeted inhibitor or antibody, or they combine target-specific blockers with classical cytotoxic drugs. Moreover, therapeutic efficiency may be further increased by using inhibitors that bind covalently instead of reversibly by hydrogen bonds to their respective substrates and thus permanently neutralise the target. Such second-generation, irreversible, multi-specific kinase inhibitors are currently in clinical development (see chapter by Solca et al.).

In summary, the recent developments in targeted therapy for breast cancer and of other neoplastic diseases have already considerably improved cancer treatment. Moreover, this era is characterized by an intense, fast and bi-directional flow of knowledge between basic science and clinical application. This type of research is growing very rapidly and has created an entirely new field of research known as "translational research", which is located right at the interface between basic science and clinical medicine. Milestone achievements during the last decade suggest that we are currently just at the beginning of a revolutionary and exciting era of cancer research, which almost certainly will tremendously improve future options for diagnosis, classification, individualisation and treatment of cancer.

Vienna, Austria

Maria Sibilia
Christoph C. Zielinski
Rupert Bartsch
Thomas W. Grunt

Reference

1. Jordan CV (1988) The development of tamoxifen for breast cancer therapy: a tribute lto the late Arthur L. Walpole. Breast Cancer Res Treat 11:197–209

Contents

The EGFR/ErbB Family in Breast Cancer: From Signalling to Therapy

Wolfgang J. Köstler and Yosef Yarden

Abstract Despite extensive diagnostic and therapeutic efforts, breast cancer remains the second leading cause of female cancer mortality in affluent countries. Because receptor tyrosine kinases of the *Epidermal Growth Factor Receptor* [EGFR, also ErbB] family are potent gatekeepers of cell fate decisions, their aberrations rank among the most frequent oncogenic insults in breast cancers. Although monoclonal antibodies and kinase inhibitors that intercept ErbB signalling can effectively inhibit progression of mammary tumours, their efficacy remains confined to a specific subset of patients. This review highlights not only the oncogenic derangements of the ErbB network in breast cancer including growth factor or receptor over-expression, but also additional loss or gain of multiple negative and positive network regulators, which override physiological mechanisms of systems control embedded in the ErbB network. We further envisage strategies to specifically target tumours at their unique network hubs, to circumvent resistance to ErbB-targeting agents and focus on network fragility exposed by oncogenic perturbations or, conversely, by targeted therapies.

1 Introduction: Breast Cancer: A Molecularly Heterogeneous Disease

The stepwise transformation of a single somatic cell with finite lifespan into a metastatic tumour is caused by multiple perturbations of regulators of cell-fate decisions [1]. The ability to sense and integrate a variety of extracellular signals and reproducibly translate these inputs into responses of defined strength, quality and duration endows the four receptor tyrosine kinases (RTKs) of the epidermal

Y. Yarden (✉)
Department of Biological Regulation, The Weizmann Institute of Science, Rehovot 76100, Israel
e-mail: yosef.yarden@weizmann.ac.il

M. Sibilia et al. (eds.), *Drugs for HER-2-positive Breast Cancer*,
Milestones in Drug Therapy, DOI 10.1007/978-3-0346-0094-1_1,

growth factor receptor (EGFR)[1] family, namely: EGFR (also denoted ERBB1), ERBB2 (Her-2/*neu*), ERBB3 and ERBB4, – with the capability to act as gatekeepers of many critical cell-fate decisions (reviewed in [2]). Accordingly, perturbations of the ErbB signalling network are heavily incriminated in tumourigenesis and metastatic progression of breast and other cancers. This chapter addresses the involvement of EGFR/ErbB signalling in the context of the emerging genomic landscape of breast cancer.

Genome-scale studies of structural and numerical DNA alterations, as well as analyses of mRNA and protein expression levels, revealed that breast cancers represent a collection of different diseases [3–7]. Each breast tumour harbours, on average, dozens of mutations, hundreds of copy number variations and thousands of differentially expressed genes compared to normal breast tissues, along with derangements in epigenetic and posttranscriptional networks, which are only beginning to be characterised. Based on recurrent patterns of such aberrations, at least five distinct breast cancer subtypes can be delineated: Luminal A and luminal B subtypes are characterised by a few chromosomal aberrations and expression profiles corresponding to oestrogen receptor signalling, fatty acid metabolism and high expression of ERBB4. In addition to these features, enhanced expression of proliferative genes attributable to activated EGFR or Her-2/*neu* signalling is observed in the luminal B subtype, and also upon emergence of endocrine resistance. The ERBB2 over-expressing subtype is characterised by over-expression of Her-2/*neu*, genes induced by this oncogene, and high level amplification of multiple other genes. The signature genes of the heterogeneous basal-like subtype are overrepresented by genes involved in cell cycle control and proliferation, stemness, genomic instability, TP53 activity and EGFR signalling. Indeed, high-level EGFR amplification may represent the pathognomic oncogenic insult of basal-like tumours with metaplastic histologic features [8]. In contrast, the biology of the rare normal-like subtype remains poorly understood.

2 Anatomy of the ErbB Network (see Fig. 1)

2.1 The Receptors and Cognate Growth Factors

With the exception of Her-2/*neu*, the generic receptor activation mechanism entails growth factor binding to the extracellular receptor portion. Eleven stimulatory polypeptide ligands with distinct receptor specificity and affinity[2] are released

[1]Official Entrez Gene symbols and full gene names are given for all protein components mentioned in this review. ERBB2 is referred to as Her-2/*neu*, whenever protein functions are discussed.

[2]Epidermal growth factor (EGF), transforming growth factor-alpha (TGF-alpha), betacellulin (BTC), and amphiregulin (AR) are specific ligands for ERBB-1, the neuregulins (NRG) 2, 3 and 4 bind only ERBB-4, whereas the ligand specificities of heparin-binding EGF (HB-EGF) and Epiregulin (EPR; both binding ERBB-1 and ERBB-4), Neuregulin-1 (NRG1; binding ERBB-3 and ERBB-4) and epigen (EPG; binding ERBB-1 and ERBB-3 or 4 in the presence of ERBB-2) are more relaxed.

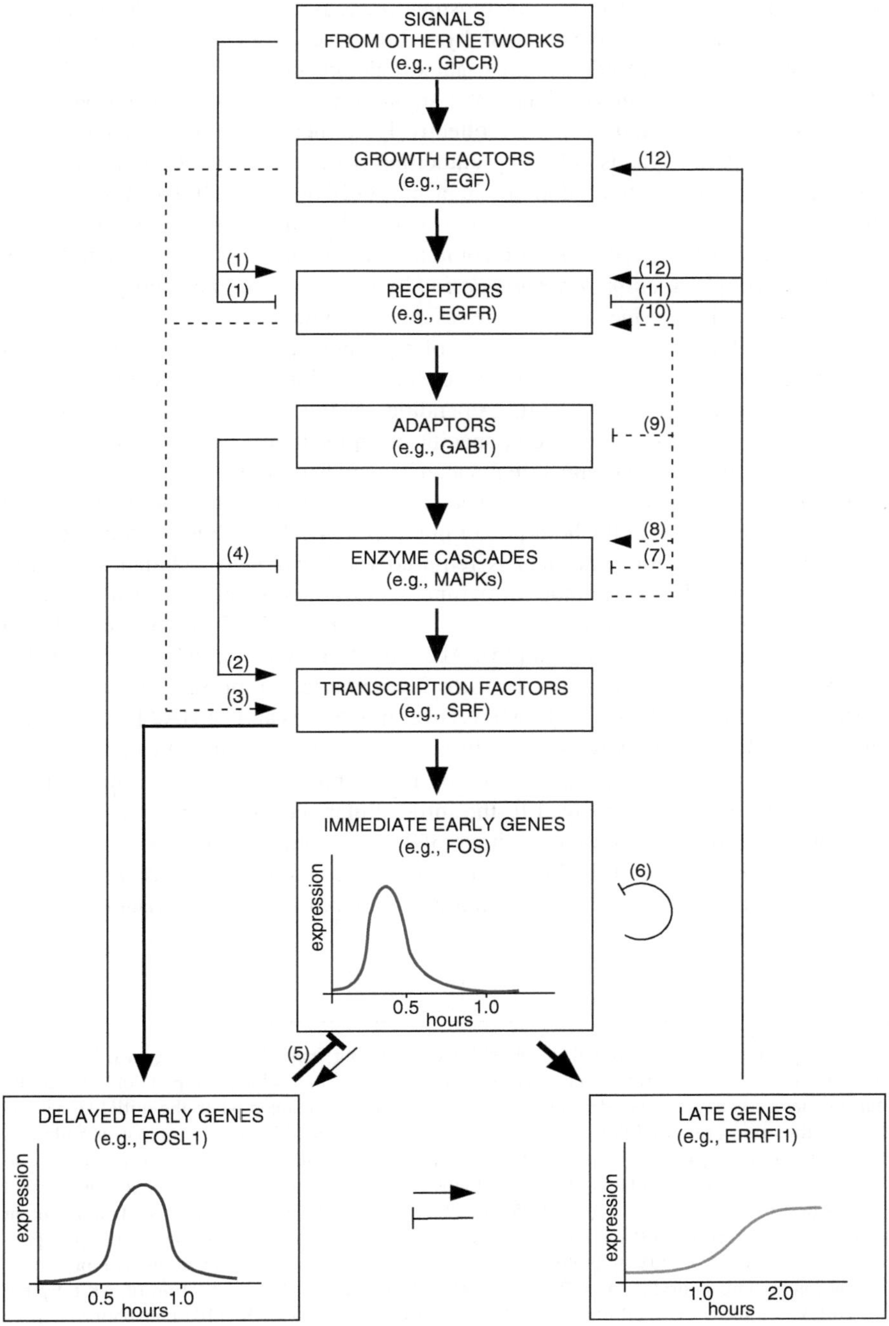

Fig. 1 Generic architecture of the ErbB network. The canonical route of propagation of signals emanating from other networks, along ligands, receptors, adaptors, enzyme cascades and transcription factors is shown along the *vertical axis*. Transcription factors launch an early

through regulated cleavage of their transmembrane precursor molecules by metalloproteases. The latter are activated by a broad set of heterologous receptors, including cytokine receptors, voltage-gated calcium channels, integrins, GPCRs (G-protein-coupled receptors) and Wnt-signalling, in response to a myriad of extracellular signals and stresses (collectively termed *receptor transactivation*) (reviewed in [9]). Ligands acting by autocrine, paracine or juxtacrine modes trap the receptor's extracellular domain in a conformation, which enables receptor dimerisation, thereby relieving the inhibition that the extracellular domain imposes on the receptor's intracellular kinase domains. Another layer of signal integration is achieved through *receptor transmodulation* by means of receptor phosphorylation on critical tyrosine, serine or threonine residues by other cellular kinases (e.g. SRC and p38 MAP kinases), or by inhibition of regulatory phosphatases [10–12]. This inter-receptor crosstalk links the ErbB network with integration of a broad variety of physical and chemical stimuli. Depending on the identity and abundance of ligands and receptors, respectively, specific receptor homo- and heterodimers are favoured, thereby determining signal specificity and strength [13].

Unlike EGFR, wild-type Her-2/*neu* is unable to form homodimers due to electrostatic repulsion at the homodimer interface [14]. Accordingly, co-expression of its heterodimerisation partners is required for Her-2/*neu*-mediated signalling [13]. Likewise, ERBB3 cannot form functional homodimers due to its inactive kinase domain. Yet, when recruited to heterodimers, ERBB3 potently couples to downstream signalling pathways [15]. Accumulating evidence suggests that ErbB receptors may also be recruited to form heteromeric complexes with other cell surface receptors, such as IGF1R, MET, several integrins and EPHA2 [16–18], thus linking ErbB signalling with an even broader set of extracellular cues.

The conformational change induced by ligand binding and dimerisation of the extracellular domains is relayed to the intracellular receptor portion, resulting in the formation of an asymmetric dimer of kinase domains: Juxtaposition of the carboxyl-terminal lobe of the kinase domain of one receptor (the *activator kinase*) upon the amino-terminal lobe of the kinase domain of its heterodimerisation partner

Fig. 1 (continued) transcriptional wave of forward-driving *immediate early genes*. This early transcriptional wave is rapidly succeeded by *delayed early genes*, which dampen both immediate early genes and enzyme cascades. Conversely, *late genes* are induced when the initial signal has ceased, thus primarily modulating the network response to repetitive or continuous stimulation. Signal amplitude, specificity and duration are fine-tuned by multiple feed-forward (1–3), and positive and negative regulatory feedback loops (4–12). Examples include (1) receptor transmodulation by other kinases, (2) STAT5B functioning as both EGFR receptor's adaptor protein and transcription factor, (3) nuclear translocation of receptors and ligands, (4) MAPK phosphatases, (5) inhibition of FOS by FOSL1, (6) autoregulatory feedback of FOS on its own promoter, (7) inhibitory phosphorylation of RAF by ERK, (8) activating phosphorylation of AKT by the mTORC2 complex, (9) inhibitory phosphorylation of GAB1 by ERK, (10) phosphorylation of EGFR by SRC, (11) inhibition of ERBB2 by ERRFI1, and (12) autocrine loops resulting in growth factor and ErbB receptor synthesis (the *receiver kinase*) induces an allosteric reorientation of the catalytic domains of the *receiver kinase* [19]. In this active asymmetric dimer conformation, the receiver kinase can transfer phosphate moieties to multiple tyrosine residues residing on the carboxyl-terminal tail of the activator. In other words, phosphorylation of ErbB receptors occurs *in trans* [19].

2.2 *Intracellular Signalling Pathways Activated by ErbB Receptors*

2.2.1 The Adaptors

Phosphorylated cytoplasmic ErbB receptor residues serve as docking sites for a broad, receptor-specific set of SRC homology 2 (SH2)- or phosphotyrosine-binding (PTB) domain-containing signalling effectors and adaptor proteins [20]. These adaptors anchor ErbB receptors to different cellular compartments, or serve as direct binders for signalling complexes linking activated receptors with canonical intracellular signalling pathways. Thus, ErbB receptors encode information through combinatorial multi-site receptor tail phosphorylation and combinations of overlapping sets of adaptor proteins [21]. For instance, instigation of cell movement and mitogenesis by EGFR is non-redundantly achieved by different phosphorylation sites [22], and elegant transgenic mouse models expressing Her-2/*neu* variants coupling to specific adaptor proteins have delineated the differential contribution of distinct signalling platforms formed with regards to tumourigenesis, proliferation, angiogenesis and metastatic outgrowth [23]. The stoichiometry and specificity of adaptor binding is also sensitive to changes in the abundance of interaction partners [21], thus linking states of increased ErbB receptor activation not only to enhanced, but also to broader signalling. For instance, phosphorylated tyrosine residues 1068 and 1086 of EGFR recruit the adaptor protein GRB2, which can bind multiple positive (e.g. SOS1) and negative (e.g. CBL) regulators of EGFR signalling, such that the net output in signalling strength and duration depends upon the abundance and activity of these proteins.

2.2.2 Signalling Pathways and Transcription Factors

The signalling pathways engaged by ErbB receptors comprise mitogen-activated protein kinase (MAPK) pathways, the phosphatidylinositol 3-kinase (PI3K), phospholipase C-γ (PLCG1) and coupling to the signal transducers and activators of transcription (STAT) family transcription factors. MAP kinases recruited by the ErbB family predominantly include the extracelluar signal-regulated kinases ERK1/2 (gene symbols: MAPK3/MAPK1), which are activated by the canonical

RAS (NRAS, HRAS and KRAS) – RAF (RAF1, BRAF and ARAF) – MEK1/2 (MAP2K1/MAP2K2) cascade, the c-Jun N-terminal kinases (JNK1/2/3), the p38 MAP kinases (isoforms MAPK14 MAPK11 MAPK12 MAPK13) and MAPK7 (also called ERK5).

The activation kinetics of these multiple sequential reactions of signal propagation from receptors to adaptors and along signalling pathways are often exponential or switch-like (*bistable*), collecting inputs over many orders of magnitude (e.g. in ligand concentrations), which can be integrated in a non-linear manner into discrete cellular outputs. The specificity and duration of the induced posttranslational modifications are integrated into discrete profiles of activity and kinetics of a much more limited set of initial transcription factors. For instance, upon nuclear translocation, ERK1 and ERK2 phosphorylate and activate the transcription factors ELK1, SP1 and multiple E2F and AP-1 transcription factors, whereas ERK5 activates MYC, FOS and serum/glucocorticoid-regulated kinases, but the JNK pathway activates ATF2, ELK1, JUN and JUNB. Depending on the identity of these transcription factor profiles, cells launch transcriptional programmes driving such diverse cellular outputs as differentiation, proliferation, metabolism, survival and motility [24, 25].

2.2.3 Nuclear Signalling of ErbB Receptors and Ligands

Beyond instigating canonical signalling cascades, ErbB receptors, ligands and their variants, may also translocate to the nucleus, where they can participate in transcriptional regulation [26–33]. Accordingly, nuclear accumulation of ErbB receptors may be associated with an adverse prognosis in patients with breast cancer [27, 28, 34–36]. It has further been argued that the synergism of ErbB-targeting agents and ionising radiation or DNA-damage inducing chemotherapeutics may critically depend upon the abrogation of nuclear ErbB signalling [37, 38].

3 ErbB Signalling as a Robust Information Relay System

3.1 From Linear Pathways to Scale-Free Feedback-Controlled Networks

The evolvement of ErbB signalling from a primordial cascade of a single ligand–receptor pair in the nematode *C. elegans* to a richly interwoven network bestowed the ErbB system of higher eukaryotes with several selective advantages: Simultaneous sensing and integration of multiple inputs allow for processing of more complex signals than concentration gradients of a single ligand (*network specification*). Moreover, functional *redundancy* of groups of signalling components (*modules*) and their rich interconnections, including feedback circuitries (Fig. 1), confer functional stability, which ensures fail-safe operation in case of perturbations in individual components or modules (*robustness*) [39]. For instance, all ErbB receptors directly or indirectly couple to the MAPK and PI3K pathways with distinct potency and outcome (*co-option*). Such *modularity*, together with the rich interconnections within and between modules, and the ability to adapt to new environmental conditions by changing the strength of their interconnections allow for network *plasticity* (also *adaptability*, *evolvability*) [40]. These scale-free networks are also characterised by *network hubs*, i.e. individual components that are more richly interconnected than other nodes and, therefore, critical to fail-safe network functioning.

3.2 Clinical Implications of Tumours as Robust Systems

In tumours, network hubs are perturbed at higher frequency than expected by random, suggesting that these aberrations confer specific advantages to tumour growth, and therefore may represent therapeutic targets [1]. An extreme manifestation of this network propensity translates to excessive reliance on very few hubs, i.e. *oncogene and non-oncogene addiction*, which comes at the price of creating network fragility [41, 42]. Whereas *oncogene addiction* conferred by aberrant positive regulatory components (e.g. oncogenes) or loss of function of negative regulators (e.g. tumour suppressor genes) has been extensively characterised, *non-oncogene addiction* entails overt reliance of tumours on network components, which do not harbour tumour-associated aberrations. A prototypical example for *non-oncogene addiction* of the ErbB network is represented by the extensive reliance of multiple, often mutated components (e.g. Her-2/*neu*, AKT, oestrogen receptor alpha (ESR1), as well as mutants of EGFR) on proper functioning of the molecular chaperone HSP90AA1 (heat shock protein 90 kDa, Hsp90) [43]. Hsp90 inhibitors, such as tanespimycin (17-AAG) or alvespimycin, which induce Her-2/*neu* ubiquitination by the ubiquitin ligase STUB1, resulting in proteasomal degradation of Her-2/*neu*, may overcome resistance to trastuzumab or to endocrine therapies [44–46].

Plasticity of the ErbB network allows tumours to evade pharmacological assaults, whilst remaining addicted to aberrant ErbB signalling. For instance, binding an epitope in subdomain IV of the Her-2/*neu* extracellular domain [14], trastuzumab may predominantly disrupt receptor heterodimers formed by an overexpressed Her-2/*neu* in the absence of ligands [47]. Conversely, pertuzumab, which binds the dimerisation loop of Her-2/*neu,* preferentially blocks ligand-instigated heterodimers of Her-2/*neu* [48]. In elegant preclinical and clinical studies, pertuzumab has shown efficacy in patients who failed prior trastuzumab therapy, and the combination of trastuzumab and pertuzumab exhibits synergism even after failure of both agents administered individually [48, 49].

3.3 Feedback Control of the ErbB Network

Network-intrinsic signal enhancers and attenuators allow response to weak stimuli (amplification), define the kinetics, amplitude and duration of signal activity and appropriately integrate the output to prolonged or repetitive stimuli. Moreover, feedback circuits act as signal linearisers that maintain output reproducibility in face of stochastic fluctuations of concentrations of individual network components, aberrant proteins or other factors that augment noise (*buffering, tolerance*) [50].

3.3.1 Early Feedback Regulation

Immediate signal-attenuation is achieved within minutes by pre-existing machineries that act primarily by inducing compartimentalization and posttranslational modifications of signalling components: These include receptor dephosphorylation by phosphatases, inhibitory phosphorylation within signalling modules and conjugation of activated receptors to ubiquitin and ubiquitin-like proteins, thereby routing them to the degradative lysosomal or proteosomal machineries. Importantly, ErbB receptors are not unique substrates for receptor proximal signal attenuators. For instance, EGFR and MET, the hepatocyte growth factor receptor, are controlled by a highly similar set of signal attenuating phosphatases and are both substrates for the ubiquitin ligase CBL, thus linking defects in these signal attenuators to unrestrained signalling by multiple RTKs [51]. Importantly, the mechanisms of immediate feedback regulation are also richly exploited by tumours to escape pharmacological assaults. For instance, buffering against incomplete inhibition of EGFR and/or Her-2/*neu* activity by kinase inhibitor therapy may occur via a shift in the phosphorylation–dephosphorylation equilibrium of ERBB3: Uncoupling of an AKT-dependent negative regulatory feedback mechanism enhances the translocation of ERBB3 from the cytoplasm to the plasma membrane, where it is available to form heterodimers – a mechanism which may be overcome by irreversible kinase inhibitors and by combining inhibitors of Her-2/*neu* and AKT [47, 52].

3.3.2 Late Feedback Regulation of Transcription

A later, broader set of signal modulators is transcriptionally induced after ErbB stimulation, and comprises positive and negative regulators of the signalling network (Fig. 1). This includes autoregulatory loops in which protein products of forward-driving *immediate early genes* (e.g. FOS) serve as transcriptional repressors at their own promoters [53]. Subsequent up-regulation of *delayed early genes,* which include transcriptional repressors and RNA-binding proteins, confines the temporal activity of *immediate early genes*. For instance, the transcriptional repressors FOSL1, KLF2 and JUNB succeed the rapid induction of the forward driving AP-1 components FOS and JUN, and RNA-binding proteins encoded by *delayed early genes*, such as ZFP36 and TIAL1, destabilise transcripts encoding for components of the AP1 complex [24, 53]. Not surprisingly, immediate early and delayed early genes regulating the ErbB system are frequently perturbed in breast and in other tumours, and their aberrations are linked to patients' prognosis [24].

3.3.3 Late Feedback Regulation of ErbB Signalling

Delayed early genes also comprise inhibitors of ErbB-induced downstream signalling cascades, such as the MAPK phosphatases (MKPs, also known as dual-specifity phosphastases, DUSPs). A later wave of transcription encodes for both positive and negative regulators that mostly act in a more receptor-proximal way. These delayed negative regulators are induced after the initial stimulus has ceased, thus they primarily attenuate the response of the ErbB system to repetitive stimulation. For instance, LRIG1, which associates with the extracellular domains of multiple receptors and recruits CBL to tag receptors for degradation [54], is frequently under-expressed in breast cancer, and its loss enhances tumourigenesis in ERBB2 transgenic mice [55]. ERRFI1 (also MIG6, RALT), another transcriptionally induced feedback inhibitor of the ErbB network, inhibits several pathways components downstream of ErbB receptors, and also directly binds to the kinase domains of EGFR, Her-2/*neu* and ERBB4, quenching their function as both activator and receiver kinases [56]. ERFFI1 under-expression, often due to genomic loss of the 1p36 region, frequently occurs in Her-2/*neu* over-expressing breast tumours, enhances their aggressiveness and promotes their resistance to targeted therapies, such as trastuzumab [57]. *De novo* transcription and rapid translocation of pre-existing Sprouty proteins (SPRY1, SPRY2) to early endosomes and to the plasma membrane are induced by RAS-MAPK signalling [58]. Sprouty proteins predominantly inhibit the activation of RAS and RAF1 as well as intercept EGFR ubiquitination and internalisation [59, 60]. SPRY1 and SPRY2 exhibit decreased expression in many mammary tumours, and their loss is accompanied by enhanced tumourigenic potential in vitro and in xenograft models [61].

In addition, microRNAs (miRs), short non-coding RNA molecules that bind to the 3′-untranslated regions of mRNAs to induce their translational repression and/or degradation, emerge as critical pre-existing and feedback-induced regulators of ErbB signalling. These molecules frequently exhibit aberrant expression attributable to epigenetic mechanisms, genomic gains or losses and to alterations in processing of their precursors (reviewed in [62]).

4 Aberrant Functions of the ErbB Network in Breast Cancer (see Fig. 2)

Because oncogenic somatic mutations of ErbB receptors are virtually absent in breast cancer [3, 6], ligand and receptor over-expression is commonly considered to be the main tumourigenic event of the ErbB system in breast cancer. Indeed,

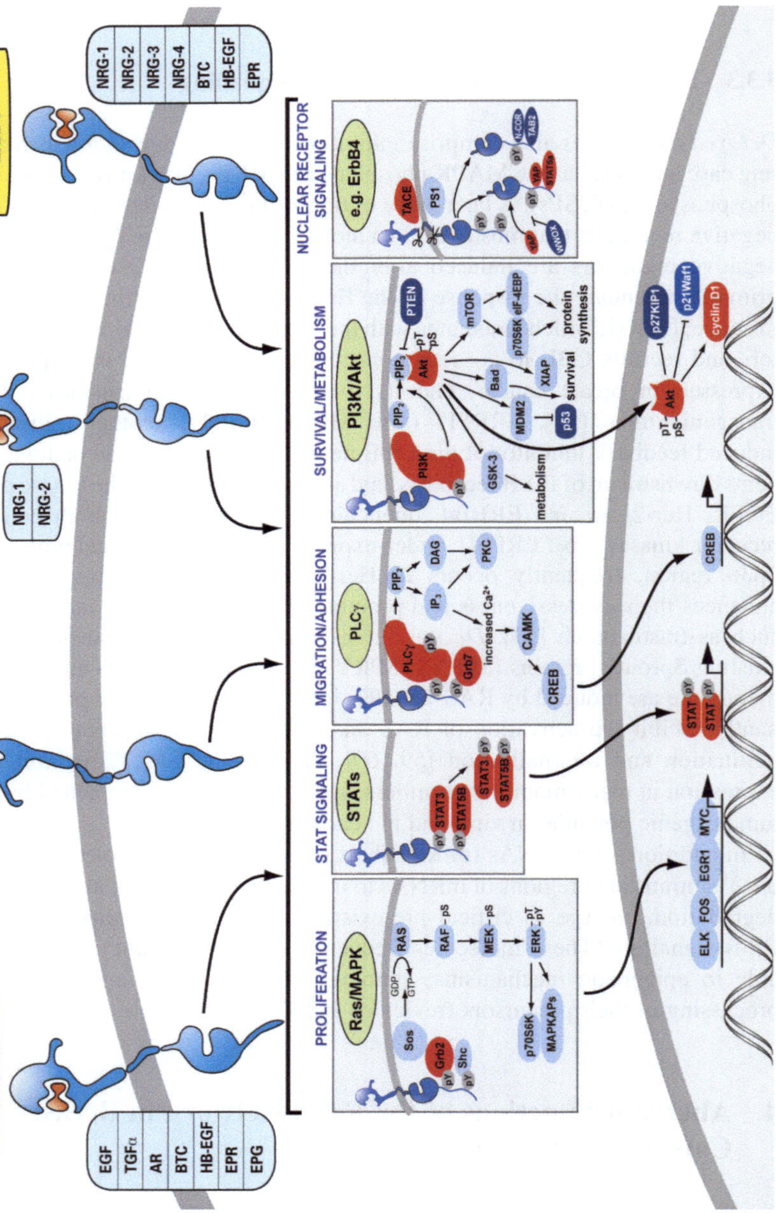

Fig. 2 (continued)

Her-2/*neu* over-expression may shift the activation/inactivation equilibrium towards higher prevalence of active receptors [63], likely by forming heterodimers [47]. However, as discussed in the following sections and as shown in Fig. 2, aberrations of the ErbB network in breast cancer predominantly include combined perturbations occurring throughout all layers of the network, including ligands, receptors, adaptor proteins and intracellular signalling cascades.

Although animal models involving conditional ERBB2 transgene expression prove that sustained expression of Her-2/*neu* is required for established metastatic tumours [64], several lines of evidence suggest that additional oncogenic hits are required: Compared to invasive ductal carinomas, approximately twice as many ductal in situ carcinomas (DCIS) over-express Her-2/*neu*, suggesting that Her-2/*neu* does not suffice for invasive outgrowth [65]. In three-dimensional cell culture models, Her-2/*neu* over-expression, but not EGFR signalling, suffices to disrupt cell polarity, increase proliferation and evade apoptosis [66]. Although Her-2/*neu* can engage multiple downstream signalling pathways involved in cell motility, including PI3K, PAK1, PTK2, RAC1 and SRC activation, heterodimerisation with EGFR and/or additional oncogenic insults, for instance enhanced transforming growth factor beta (TGFB1) signalling, are required to achieve an invasive phenotype and further support cell survival [67–70]. In transgenic mice, over-expression of wild-type human Her-2/*neu* under control of its endogenous promoter generates mammary tumours with low metastatic potential only after long latency [23]. Consistent with in vitro models, ERBB2 transgenic mice require EGFR, β-catenin (CTNNB1), and/or TGFB1 signalling and/or TP53 loss as synergistic inducers of mammary tumourigenesis and/or metastatic outgrowth [23]. Below we discuss potential collaborators of Her-2/*neu* in mammary tumourigenesis.

4.1 The Her-2/neu Amplicon

While EGFR amplification occurs in approximately 5% of breast cancer [8], amplification of a genomic region containing the ERBB2 gene on chromosome 17q12 occurs in approximately 25% of invasive breast tumours [65]. The minimum region of recurrent amplification includes the Her-2/*neu* adaptor protein GRB7

Fig. 2 (continued) ErbB receptors, their ligands and downstream signalling pathways perturbed in breast cancer. ErbB receptors activated by binding of their respective ligands (ligands are shown in *light blue boxes*) couple via adaptor proteins to intracellular signalling cascades, including MAPK, STAT transcription factors, PLC-γ and PI3K-AKT signalling. Alternately, ErbB receptors may serve as transcriptional co-regulators in the nucleus. Pathway components downstream of ErbB receptors, which frequently exhibit enhanced expression or gain-of function mutations in breast cancer, are highlighted in *red*, signal attenuators frequently lost in breast cancer are depicted in *dark blue* (reviewed below) and STARD3 (involved in endosomal vesicle trafficking). The commonly amplified region contains five additional genes, which are over-expressed along with Her-2/*neu* and constitute part of the ERBB2 gene expression signature in breast cancer [71], including PPP1R1B (protein phosphatase 1, regulatory (inhibitor) subunit 1B, also DARPP32), splice variants of which have been associated with resistance to trastuzumab, and C17ORF37 (chromosome 17 open reading frame 37, also MGC14832), which promotes migration and invasion by serving as a positive regulator of AKT phosphorylation. Furthermore, multiple genes promoting the growth of ErbB-dependent breast cancer, such as topoisomerase II, are frequently co-amplified and over-expressed along with Her-2/*neu* [7]. Importantly, ERBB2 amplification often occurs on the background of a polysomy of chromosome 17, leading to deregulation of many genes involved in breast cancer pathogenesis and treatment response (reviewed in [72, 73]).

4.2 Transcriptional Control of ErbB Receptor Expression

The gene dosage gain of a few extra copies of ERBB2 may not account for the remarkable increase in mRNA and protein levels observed in ERBB2-amplified breast tumours, suggesting the occurrence of additional mechanisms governing the increased transcription, predominantly mono-allelic, from amplified ERBB2 genes [74]. In most Her-2/neu over-expressing breast tumours, multiple transcription factors enhancing ERBB2 promoter activity (e.g. the AP-2 family of proteins, factors engaging the AP-2 complex, such as Yin Yang 1, various Ets factor family members, EGR2, ZO-1 and ZONAB) show enhanced expression or activity. In addition, these are accompanied by frequent genomic or functional loss of trans-repressors of the ERBB2 promoter, such as FOXP3, GATA4, RB1, WWOX and the Ets protein PEA [75, 76].

4.3 Variant Receptors

Her-2/*neu* over-expression is almost universally accompanied by a disproportional shift in the expression of receptor variants compared to the more abundant full length, 185 kDa, wild-type receptor. Approximately 50% of Her-2/*neu* over-expressing breast tumours exhibit enhanced expression of amino-terminally truncated Her-2/*neu* receptors lacking most of the extracellular receptor portion. These variant receptors are generated by alternative translation initiation (resulting in receptor sizes in the range of 90–120 kDa) or by ADAM10-mediated proteolytic cleavage of the extracellular domain, resulting in a 95 kDa carboxyl-terminal receptor fragment (p95) [32, 77–82]. Her-2/*neu* truncation variants exhibit constitutive activity: Some variants constitutively form receptor homodimers, undergo enhanced nuclear translocation or exhibit a significantly enhanced transforming potential in transgenic animal models [79]. Thus, more than the wild-type receptor, their expression has been associated with adverse prognosis in patients with Her-2/*neu* over-expressing breast cancers.

Importantly, all these receptor variants lack the trastuzumab-binding epitope, but remain sensitive to lapatinib [83]. Moreover, the secreted ectodomain (ECD) resulting from proteolytic receptor cleavage may bind and neutralise trastuzumab, resulting in sub-therapeutic trastuzumab serum levels in patients presenting very high ECD levels [84, 85]. Conversely, binding to an epitope near the cleavage site, trastuzumab inhibits proteolytic cleavage of Her-2/*neu* [86]. These mutual pharmacokinetic and pharmacodynamic interactions make measurement of ECD levels an ideal tool to monitor the efficacy of ongoing therapy with trastuzumab [87, 88].

Another HER-2 variant, HER2Δ16, likely generated by alternative mRNA splicing, lacks a small part of the extracellular domain and accounts for up to 9% of Her-2/*neu* transcripts in mammary tumours. HER2Δ16 constitutively forms homodimers, potently couples to downstream signalling pathways and exhibits potent transforming activity [89]. Although HER2Δ16 binds trastuzumab, the enhanced SRC kinase activity conferred by this variant interferes with plasma membrane recruitment and activation of PTEN required for trastuzumab efficacy [90]. HER2Δ16 expressing cells, however, are exquisitely sensitive to lapatinib and SRC inhibitors [91, 92].

Production of receptor variants is not limited to Her-2/*neu*. Enhanced expression of EGFRvIII, an EGFR variant lacking large parts of the extracellular ligand-binding domain encoded by exons 2–7, has been described in breast cancers [93, 94]. EGFRvIII exhibits constitutive, ligand-independent receptor and PI3K pathway activity [95], thus explaining the sensitivity of tumours expressing EGFR-vIII to combined treatment with EGFR and mTOR inhibitors and to antibodies specifically binding with EGFRvIII, but not with the wild-type receptor [96, 97]. Mammary tumours also shift the expression of ERBB4 towards cleavable isoforms, along with enhanced expression of their sheddase, ADAM17, thereby conferring tumourigenic ERBB4 activity even in the absence of ligand [36].

4.4 Ligands

Enhanced proteolytic release of AREG, HB-EGF and TGFA from breast cancer cells occurs through up-regulation or mutations of sheddases. The latter include ADAMTS1, MMP1, ADAM17 and ADAM12 [3, 98], as well as other extracellular matrix degrading enzymes. Altered expression of these components may modify tumourigenesis and metastatic outgrowth in ERBB2 transgenic mouse models (reviewed in [99]). Enhanced synthesis of the ligands predominantly results from autocrine transcriptional loops involving ligand-stimulation-mediated transcriptional induction of ligand and receptor production, boosting the autonomous growth of breast cancer [24, 25, 100]. For instance, constitutive expression of TGFA in the mammary epithelium is tumourigenic and synergises with receptor over-expression

[101]. Ligand secretion also links mammary tumours to their microenvironment. For instance, a paracrine loop involving EGF and pro-angiogenic factors produced by tumour-associated M2 macrophages acts as a chemotactic migratory stimulus required for the invasiveness of breast cancer cells in vivo whereas colony-stimulating factor-1 (CSF1) produced by tumour cells acts as potent chemoattractant for macrophages [102].

Tumour-derived ErbB ligands also suppress the expression of osteoprotegerin by osteoblasts, thereby potentiating differentiation of osteoclasts involved in the formation of bone metastases [103]. Conversely, ErbB ligands released, for instance, during healing of surgical wounds stimulate the proliferation of HER-2/*neu* over-expressing breast tumours [104, 105]. Increased ligand production is causally involved in resistance to some ErbB-targeting agents. For instance, ligand production causes resistance to cetuximab, in part by competing with antibody binding to EGFR. Likewise, ligand production in Her-2/*neu* over-expressing breast tumours increases resistance to trastuzumab by formation of ligand-mediated receptor heterodimers [106]. Moreover, increased production of alternatively spliced variant forms of TGFA and neuregulin precursors, mediating enhanced transforming ability by increased secretion, differential binding to ErbB family members or nuclear translocation, have been identified in breast cancer [107].

4.5 Adaptor Proteins and Substrates

SRC: The cytoplasmic tyrosine kinase SRC (v-src sarcoma viral oncogene homolog) acts as both an upstream activator and a substrate of ErbB family members (reviewed in [108]). Enhanced expression and activity of ErbB family members and SRC are frequently observed in breast cancer in association with adverse prognosis. SRC-induced phosphorylation of the non-autophosphorylation site on tyrosine 845 couples EGFR to the transcription factor STAT5B required for mitogenesis and DNA repair, as well as to the cytochrome *c* oxidase subunit II, resulting in inhibition of apoptosis by interference of cytochrome *c* release from mitochondria. SRC also enhances coupling of EGFR to STAT and JNK proteins, the regulatory subunit of PI3K, and SRC-mediated phosphorylation of EGFR enhances the receptor's interaction with SRC itself.

Receptor trans-modulation by SRC also links the EGFR to signals emanating from integrins and GPCRs, and signals from ErbB receptors in turn regulate integrin assembly and function required for tumourigenesis and metastatic outgrowth [108, 109]. Importantly, this transmodulation-mediated recruitment of EGFR to signalling complexes, independent of its kinase activity, may account for resistance of EGFR over-expressing mammary tumours to EGFR-targeting kinase inhibitors [110]. Recent studies also implicate the EGFR-SRC axis in resistance to pathway inhibitors downstream of both kinases: For instance, rapamycin-induced EGFR activation via SRC has been implicated in resistance to this mTOR inhibitor [111]. Her-2/*neu* promotes SRC synthesis and stability, and physically associates with SRC [112]. Indeed, SRC activity is crucially involved in Her-2/*neu*-mediated anchorage-independent growth, survival, motility, invasion and metastases in cell cultures and in animal models [112, 113]. Conversely, SRC also acts upstream of Her-2/*neu* by enhancing tyrosine phosphorylation and heterodimer formation of Her-2/*neu* with ERBB3, and by enhancing the coupling of p85 to receptor complexes, SRC instigates increased basal and/or neuregulin-induced activation [114]. SRC also directly phosphorylates multiple substrates of the ErbB pathway, including focal adhesion kinase, cortactin, PI3K and STAT proteins (reviewed in [115]), thus fine-tuning their activity. Moreover, association with SRC also links oestrogen and progesterone receptor signalling to activation of the RAS-MAPK pathway [116].

GRB7: The adaptor protein GRB7 (growth factor receptor-bound protein 7) is co-amplified, over-expressed and forms a physical complex with HER-2/*neu* in ERBB2-amplified breast cancers, where it facilitates phosphorylation of Her-2/*neu* and its interaction with PLCG1 (phospholipase c-γ1) and AKT, thereby enhancing tumourigenesis in xenograft models [117]. GRB7 can also bind ERBB3 and ERBB4, coupling ErbB receptors to Shc [118]. Through its interaction with calmodulin and focal adhesion kinase, GRB7 also enhances cellular motility and mediates anti-oestrogen resistance by a yet unidentified mechanism.

Phospholipase C-γ1. PLCG1 exhibits enhanced expression and activity in the majority of EGFR and/or Her-2/*neu* over-expressing mammary tumours [119]. In addition to regulating cell motility via indirect effects on the activity of actin-modifying proteins, PLCG1 hydrolyses phosphatidylinositol (4,5) bisphosphate (PIP_2) into the second messengers inositol-1,4,5-trisphosphate (IP_3) and diacylglycerol (DAG). IP_3 is important for intracellular calcium mobilisation and for the activation of calcium/calmodulin-dependent protein kinases and phosphatases. DAG serves as a co-factor for calcium in activation of protein kinase C, which, in turn, activates MAPK and c-Jun NH2-terminal kinases.

GRB2. Through binding of SHC, GAB1, CBL, TNK2 and SOS, the adaptor protein GRB2 (growth factor receptor-bound protein 2) links ErbB receptors to the RAS-MAPK pathway, the p85 regulatory subunit of PI3K and to the endocytic machinery [120]. GRB2, located on chromosome 17q24-q25, is frequently over-expressed along with the phosphatase PTPN6 in mammary tumours [121].

GAB2. The scaffolding adaptor GAB2 (Grb2-associated binding protein 2) maps to a region (11q13-14) amplified in approximately 15% and over-expressed in almost 50% of mammary tumours [122]. The hyperactivation of the RAS-MAPK pathway resulting from GAB2 over-expression and its interaction with the phosphatase PTPN11 enhances breast carcinogenesis and metastatic outgrowth in ERBB2 transgenic mice [122].

STAT3. The transcription factor STAT3 links ErbB-driven mammary tumours to the microenvironment. Constitutive activation of STAT3 alone is weakly tumourigenic, but it occurs in a large fraction of human breast tumours [123]. In ERBB2-driven transgenic mouse models, transcriptional programmes launched by STAT3 instigate an inflammatory and angiogenic acute phase response, which boosts metastatic outgrowth [124].

5 Beyond Receptors and Adaptors: Global Aberrations in ErbB- Regulated Pathways in Breast Cancer

Beyond the aberrations of the PI3K pathway and the phosphatases discussed below, multiple less abundant driver and passenger mutations of the ErbB system can be observed at lower frequency in breast cancer: These affect GAB1, IRS2, BRAF, KRAS, several MAP kinases (e.g. MAP3K6, MAPK13, PRKAA2), actin organisers such as CDC42-binding protein kinases, regulators and effectors of RHO GTPases (e.g. ARHGEF4, ARHGAP25, ROCK1, PKN1) and calcium/calmodulin-dependent kinases, as well as mTOR signalling components and ribosomal protein S6 kinases (e.g. PRKAA2, RPS6KA3, RPS6KA4, RPS6KC1) [3, 4, 6]. Moreover, multiple signalling modules exhibit enhanced expression due to gene amplification at lower frequency (e.g. AKT2, RPS6KB1, PTK6), and critically modify the responsiveness to ErbB targeting agents, such as trastuzumab [7, 125, 126]. Furthermore, multiple alterations of posttranscriptional processes modify the transforming role of ErbB alterations in mammary tumours. For instance, alternatively spliced isoforms of vasodilator-stimulated phosphoprotein (VASP) family members involved in actin remodelling co-operate with EGF signalling to promote metastases in breast cancer [127]. Below, we review frequent alterations depicted in Fig. 2 that impact on major signalling pathways at several locations, potentially creating synergistic effects for tumourigenesis, metastatic growth and resistance to pharmacological interventions.

5.1 Aberrations in the PI3K–AKT Pathway

Amplification and mutations of PI3K occur in approximately 25% of mammary tumours, particularly those characterised by ESR1 expression and/or ERBB2 amplification. Activating point mutations of PI3K cluster in hotspots within the kinase and helical domains of the catalytic subunit (PIK3CA) [128] or, less frequently, encompass the regulatory PI3K subunits [3, 6]. PI3K mutations confer constitutive phosphorylation of AKT on residues T308 and S473, resulting in increased phosphorylation of the transcription factors FOXO1 and FOXO3, whereas other AKT targets are not consistently affected [129]. Thus, oncogenic mutations of PI3K are not biologically equivalent to the frequent loss of PTEN discussed below [130].

The 3′ phosphoinositide-dependent protein kinase 1 (PDPK1) links phosphoinositides produced by PI3K to AKT activation. PDPK1 is frequently amplified in breast cancer and the majority of tumours exhibit enhanced expression of this kinase – particularly those with Her-2/*neu* over-expression. Whilst not oncogenic by itself, PDPK1 over-expression enhances the transforming potential of upstream perturbations [131, 132]. In preclinical models, novel compounds inhibiting PDPK1 show single agent and synergistic activity with trastuzumab, even in tumours resistant to trastuzumab [133]. Conversely, constitutive AKT1 activation by mutations occurs at much lower frequency in breast cancer (1–8%) [130, 134]. AKT1 mutations lead to phosphorylation and subsequent destruction of TSC2, which promotes tumour survival and proliferation, whilst diminishing RHOA-GTPase activity and transcriptional networks required for cell motility and invasion [134–136]. Interestingly, constitutive AKT2 activation promotes cell invasion, but inhibits tumour growth [137].

5.2 *Perturbations of the Endocytic Machinery in ErbB-Driven Mammary Tumours*

Clathrin-mediated and clathrin-independent endocytic mechanisms represent the main mediators of immediate sequestration of activated ErbB receptors from the plasma membrane (reviewed in [138, 139]). This is achieved by multiple post-translational modifications of signalling complexes, clathrin assembly proteins and the entire endocytic machinery. Covalent tagging of signalling complexes with ubiquitin and ubiquitin-like moieties (e.g. NEDD8) couples receptors to ubiquitin-binding domain containing endosomal sorting proteins. The journey of internalised receptors along the endocytic route from early to late endosomes culminates in signal attenuation and sorting for intracellular degradation in the multivesicular body. Endosomal sorting of EGFR critically depends upon its persistent ligand binding, phosphorylation, ubiquitination and continued association with the ubiquitin E3 ligase CBL, which prevents receptor recycling from early and late endosomal compartments back to the plasma membrane [140]. Aside from receptors, CBL also ubiquitinates adapator proteins and endocytic adaptors, thereby promoting internalisation and degradative sorting of whole signalling complexes.

Beyond functioning as a mere desensitisation process, endocytic trafficking and recycling of receptor cargo is also crucially required for maintenance of matrix adhesion and cell–cell contacts and, thereby, for epithelial polarity and cell migration. Indeed, the polarity-maintaining endocytic routing is perturbed by oncogenic ErbB signalling in many tumours – predominantly by acting on polarity genes of the Par (partitioning-defective) family. EGFR enhances tight junction assembly by inducing SRC-mediated phosphorylation of PARD3, whereas Her-2/*neu* disrupts apical–basal cell polarity by associating with the PARD6–PRKCI complex [141, 142]. EGFR also regulates endocytosis of cadherins by coupling to ARF6 via its GEF, IQSEQ1, which is frequently over-expressed in highly invasive breast tumours [143]. In addition, the endocytic machinery compartmentalises signalling of ErbB receptors, allowing them to engage in signalling complexes that are qualitatively distinct from those formed at the plasma membrane [50, 144].

5.2.1 Evading the CBL Hub

To maintain malignant phenotypes, oncogenic perturbations in ErbB signalling must evade or perturb the endocytic machinery or be accompanied by defects in key endocytic regulators. While over-expression of receptors can saturate the binding capacity of both clathrin-coated pits and endosomal adaptors, further prolonging half-life of active receptors [145], overcoming the negative regulatory effect of CBL represents another key event required for tumourigenesis by the ErbB network. For instance, activated SRC phosphorylates clathrin and dynamin [146], resulting in enhanced EGFR internalisation, whilst SRC-mediated phosphorylation of the ubiquitin ligase CBL results in CBL's autoubiquitination and proteasomal degradation, thus promoting EGFR recycling [147]. The net effect is enhanced membranal and endosomal signalling of EGFR in the absence of EGFR degradation. As CBL and its family members, CBLB and CBLC, have multiple substrates in addition to EGFR, including other growth factor receptors, cytokine receptors, hormone receptors and integrins [148], perturbations of CBL result in unbalanced partitioning of multiple cargos between the route leading to lysosomal degradation and the alternative recycling route. Indeed, CBL knockout mice exhibit hyperplasia of multiple tissues, including the mammary epithelium [149].

Autocrine loops involving overproduction of growth factors that lose receptor affinity in the mildly acidic early endosomes, such as TGFA, EPGN and HBEGF, also evade the regulatory role of CBL: Dissociation of receptor–ligand complexes decreases phosphorylation of endosomal EGFR and its association with CBL, resulting in enhanced receptor recycling [150, 151]. The EGFRvIII variant is poorly downregulated because of its decreased phosphorlyation on the CBL docking site at tyrosine 1045, and its constitutive association with HSP90 [152]. Similarly, EGFR transmodulation may alter the endocytic fate of the receptor [12].

Unlike EGFR, Her-2/*neu* poorly internalises or couples to the degradative endocytic machinery, but readily recycles, thereby enhancing protein levels and prolonging the signalling of its heterodimerization partners [13, 153–155]. Accordingly, increased expression of Her-2/*neu* or ligands promoting the formation of Her-2/*neu* containing heterodimers, such as EREG and EPGN, promotes the transforming role of its heterodimerisation partners [150, 153, 156].

5.2.2 Aberrations in Endocytic Components

The CDC42 guanine nucleotide exchange factor (GEF) called ARHGEF7 (also betaPix, Cool-1) is frequently over-expressed and/or activated by EGFR and SRC in breast cancer [157]. The resulting formation of a CDC42/ARHGEF7/CBL complex, which sequesters CBL from EGFR, diminishes EGFR ubiquitination and downregulation [158]. Cortactin (CTTN), an actin-binding protein, is over-expressed due to amplification of the 11q13 region in about 13% of primary breast carcinomas [159] and inhibits CBL-mediated down-regulation of EGFR [160] in multiple ways: Impaired tyrosine phosphorylation of CBL and association with EGFR occur through enhanced SRC activity, and activation of CDC42 via the exchange protein FGD1 enhances the formation of the CDC42/ARHGEF7/CBL complex [160]. Other examples of impaired ErbB receptor endocytosis in breast cancer involve LIMK1, the actin adaptor HIP1, the ubiquitin E3 ligases WWP1, ITCH, NRDP1 and NEDD4, and the ubiquitin-binding protein TSG101.

5.3 *Perturbations of Protein and Lipid Phosphatases Acting at and Downstream to ErbB Receptors*

Along with MAPK phosphatases acting on signalling pathways downstream of ErbB receptors, cytoplasmic and plasma-membrane-anchored tyrosine and lipid phosphatases critically define the window of receptor activation in different cellular compartments (reviewed in [161]). The activity of protein tyrosine phosphatases is negatively regulated by oxidation of their active site cysteine residue by H_2O_2 produced by oxidative stress and by some tyrosine kinase inhibitors. Likewise, phosphorylation on serine, threonine or tyrosine residues differentially modulates the activity of phosphatases, and links their activity to inputs from tyrosine kinases and GPCRs [162].

Phosphatases that enhance ErbB signalling, and frequently exhibit increased expression and/or activity in breast cancer, include PTPN11 (protein tyrosine phosphatase, non-receptor type 11, also SHP2), PTPRE (protein tyrosine phosphatase, receptor type, E) and PTPN1 (protein tyrosine phosphatase, non-receptor type 1, also PTP1B). Conversely, protein phosphatases, which quench the activity of ErbB receptors, such as PTPN13 (protein tyrosine phosphatase, non-receptor type 13, also PTP1E, PTPL1), PTPN6 (protein tyrosine phosphatase, non-receptor type 6, also SHP-1), PTPRF (protein tyrosine phosphatase, receptor type, F, also PTP-LAR) and PTPRJ (protein tyrosine phosphatase, receptor type, J, also DEP-1) are frequently lost or exhibit decreased activity in breast cancer. Likewise, the lipid phosphatase INPPL (inositol polyphosphate phosphatase-like 1, also SHIP2), which enhances EGFR levels by interfering with degradative sorting of EGFR in early endosomes, is frequently over-expressed in mammary tumours [163]. PTEN (phosphatase and tensin homolog deleted on chromosome 10) dephosphorylates phosphoinositide substrates, dephosphorylates proteins on serine, threonine and tyrosine residues and executes multiple functions independent of its phosphatase activity. PTEN hydrolyses phosphatidylinositol-3,4,5-trisphosphate (PIP_3) to generate phosphatidylinositol (4,5) bi-phosphate (PIP_2), which functionally antagonises the activating function of PI3K towards PDPK1 and AKT [164] (Fig. 2). In addition to regulating multiple other cytoplasmic substrates, PTEN also dephosphorylates RTKs, thus acting both upstream and downstream of ErbB receptors. Indeed, enhanced activation of ERBB3 and IGF1R due to PTEN loss may contribute to endocrine resistance of breast cancer, and a kinase inhibitor, lapatinib, may decrease ERBB3 phosphorylation in PTEN-deficient tumours by sequestering Her-2/*neu* into inactive heterodimers with EGFR [165]. In the nucleus, PTEN serves as a transcriptional repressor of multiple genes involved in cell growth and metastases, and as an essential gatekeeper of genome integrity (reviewed in [166]). For instance, PTEN regulates arrest at the G1 phase of the cell cycle by down-regulating cyclin D1 transcription, by preventing the AKT-induced cytoplasmic sequestration of the cyclin-dependent kinase inhibitor CDKN1B (also $p27^{Kip1}$) and by enhancing $p27^{Kip1}$ transcription via forkhead transcription factors, which otherwise undergo inhibitory phosphorylation by AKT. Indeed, $p27^{Kip1}$ acts as an essential mediator of growth arrest induced by ErbB targeting agents: Together, p27^{Kip1} loss and/or over-expression of cyclin D1 occur in 50% of breast cancers, and both are associated with therapeutic resistance to ErbB-targeting agents [167–169]. In ERBB2 transgenic mouse models, p27^{Kip1} haploinsufficiency accelerates mammary tumourigenesis [170].

In up to 50% of sporadic mammary tumours, PTEN haploinsufficiency or loss occurs by multiple, non-exclusive mechanisms, including mutations encoding unstable or catalytically inactive PTEN, deletions and epigenetic silencing, lack-of-function PTEN splice variants and posttranscriptional downregulation by micro-RNAs. Moreover, PTEN activity, protein stability, localisation and interactions are regulated by multiple post-translational modifications, which link PTEN function to multiple intracellular signalling pathways. For instance, Her-2/*neu* over-expressing mammary tumours activate SRC to phosphorylate PTEN, sequestering it from its active site at the plasma membrane [90]. Indeed, the ability to revert this inhibition is critically relevant to the clinical efficacy of therapeutics targeting EGFR or Her-2/*neu* in breast and in other tumours, because hypersensitivity of the PI3K pathway resulting from complete loss of PTEN expression has been associated with resistance to trastuzumab and to EGFR tyrosine kinase inhibitors, but less so with resistance to lapatinib which more efficiently shuts down phosphorylation of all ErbB family members and sequesters them from associating with IGF1R [90, 165, 171–177].

5.4 Implications to Targeting ErbB Receptors and Their Downstream Pathways

While constitutive activation of multiple network components mitigates the effects of ErbB-targeting drugs, inhibitors of downstream signalling pathways exhibit only modest and transient single-agent activity in breast cancer treatment. Because multiple negative regulatory feedback loops are disengaged by treatment with pathway inhibitors alone, rationally designed combinations of anti-ErbB agents with pathway inhibitors emerge as promising new therapeutic regimens, despite limited activity of individual agents. From a systems biology perspective, the design of such combinations requires thorough understanding of the architecture, of the targeted network: At clinically achievable drug dosages, drug efficacy decreases substantially if a functional negative feedback loop inactivates a component upstream of a drug target, whereas drugs acting outside of the feedback loop may result in more pronounced pathway inhibition [178]. A prototypical example includes rapamycin and rapalogs, which predominantly inhibit the mTOR complex 1 (mTORC1, formed by mTOR, RAPTOR, MLST8, and AKT1S1) involved in protein synthesis. mTORC1 inhibition alleviates the feedback inhibition of the upstream activator IRS1 and of PI3K, mediated by the mTOR target ribosomal protein S6 p70 kinase, and results in enhanced activation of both, the PI3K–AKT and the RAS–MAPK pathways [179–181]. Moreover, the mTOR complex 2 (formed by mTOR, RICTOR,

MAPKAP1, PRR5 and MLST8), which phosphorylates AKT, thus causing sensitisation to upstream signals, is not inhibited by rapamycin in most cell lines (reviewed in [182]). Thus, due to the dampening of feedback inhibition circuits, the supersensitivity of ERBB2 amplified, PTEN lacking or PI3K-mutated tumours to inhibitors of AKT and mTOR is only transient, resulting in moderate efficacy of these agents in patients with breast cancer [183, 184]. In combination with ErbB – or IGF1R – targeting agents, however, inhibitors of PI3K, AKT and/or mTOR can restore or enhance sensitivity to trastuzumab or to lapatinib, respectively, resulting in exquisite synergism in both preclinical models and in initial clinical trials [44, 45, 83, 90, 174, 184–190].

Combining PI3K–AKT–mTOR inhibitors with those of other pathways represents another promising strategy: For instance, despite evidence of target inhibition, MEK inhibitors have shown very limited efficacy in patients with breast cancer [191], likely because inhibition of MEK attenuates a negative MEK–EGFR–PI3K feedback loop [192]. Accordingly, combined inhibition of mTOR or EGFR and MEK has shown synergistic activity in several cancer xenograft models [181]. In a different signalling context, namely tumours carrying B-RAF mutations, anti-EGFR antibodies were identified as synergistic combination partners of the kinase inhibitor sorafenib [193]. This is analogous to the aforementioned synergistic combinations of ErbB-targeting agents with SRC inhibitors or with HSP90 inhibitors.

6 Outlook

Our improved understanding of the regulation of the ErbB network, as well as the relevant oncogenic perturbations, has already enabled the design of effective therapeutic agents to treat breast cancer. As highlighted in this chapter, besides perturbations in ErbB receptors, mammary tumours harbour multiple downstream aberrations, which likely enhance tumourigenic potential and modify response to therapeutic agents. Rationally designed targeted therapies will have to take this multiplicity of oncogenic perturbations into account, as well as identify fragile hubs specific to individual tumours. Such endeavours entail high-throughput approaches able to identify perturbations and their collective effects, along with analytical and pharmacological strategies that can generate safe and effective interventions. Since different oncogenic perturbations result in discrete transcriptional signatures, deconstruction of pathways into ensembles of modules can already predict drug sensitivity [194, 195]. Similarly, mathematical modelling of reactions of the ErbB network, based upon network kinetics measured *in vitro*, holds promise for the prediction of response to individual or combined therapeutic perturbations [177, 196, 197]. Finally, such approaches may also resolve mechanisms of acquired resistance to ErbB-targeted therapies, and delineate strategies to prevent or overcome adaptive resistance.

Acknowledgements We thank members of our lab team for insightful comments. YY is the incumbent of the Harold and Zelda Goldenberg Professorial Chair and W.J.K. is supported by a PhD Track for Specialist MDs fellowship of the The Linda and Michael Jacobs Charitable Trust. Our work is supported by research grants from the U.S. National Cancer Institute (NCI; CA072981), the Israel Science Foundation, Dr. Miriam and Sheldon G. Adelson Medical Research Foundation and the German-Israel Foundation.

References

1. Hanahan D, Weinberg RA (2000) The hallmarks of cancer. Cell 100:57–70
2. Yarden Y, Sliwkowski MX (2001) Untangling the ErbB signalling network. Nat Rev Mol Cell Biol 2:127–137
3. Greenman C, Stephens P, Smith R, Dalgliesh GL, Hunter C, Bignell G, Davies H, Teague J, Butler A, Stevens C et al (2007) Patterns of somatic mutation in human cancer genomes. Nature 446:153–158
4. Sjoblom T, Jones S, Wood LD, Parsons DW, Lin J, Barber TD, Mandelker D, Leary RJ, Ptak J, Silliman N et al (2006) The consensus coding sequences of human breast and colorectal cancers. Science 314:268–274
5. Perou CM, Sorlie T, Eisen MB, van de Rijn M, Jeffrey SS, Rees CA, Pollack JR, Ross DT, Johnsen H, Akslen LA et al (2000) Molecular portraits of human breast tumours. Nature 406:747–752
6. Wood LD, Parsons DW, Jones S, Lin J, Sjoblom T, Leary RJ, Shen D, Boca SM, Barber T, Ptak J et al (2007) The genomic landscapes of human breast and colorectal cancers. Science 318:1108–1113
7. Neve RM, Chin K, Fridlyand J, Yeh J, Baehner FL, Fevr T, Clark L, Bayani N, Coppe JP, Tong F et al (2006) A collection of breast cancer cell lines for the study of functionally distinct cancer subtypes. Cancer Cell 10:515–527
8. Reis-Filho JS, Milanezi F, Carvalho S, Simpson PT, Steele D, Savage K, Lambros MB, Pereira EM, Nesland JM, Lakhani SR et al (2005) Metaplastic breast carcinomas exhibit EGFR, but not HER2, gene amplification and overexpression: immunohistochemical and chromogenic in situ hybridization analysis. Breast Cancer Res 7:R1028–R1035
9. Fischer OM, Hart S, Gschwind A, Ullrich A (2003) EGFR signal transactivation in cancer cells. Biochem Soc Trans 31:1203–1208
10. Yamauchi T, Ueki K, Tobe K, Tamemoto H, Sekine N, Wada M, Honjo M, Takahashi M, Takahashi T, Hirai H et al (1997) Tyrosine phosphorylation of the EGF receptor by the kinase Jak2 is induced by growth hormone. Nature 390:91–96
11. Frank SJ (2008) Mechanistic Aspects of Crosstalk Between GH and PRL and ErbB Receptor Family Signaling. J Mammary Gland Biol Neoplasia 13:119–129
12. Zwang Y, Yarden Y (2006) p38 MAP kinase mediates stress-induced internalization of EGFR: implications for cancer chemotherapy. EMBO J 25:4195–4206
13. Pinkas-Kramarski R, Soussan L, Waterman H, Levkowitz G, Alroy I, Klapper L, Lavi S, Seger R, Ratzkin BJ, Sela M et al (1996) Diversification of Neu differentiation factor and epidermal growth factor signaling by combinatorial receptor interactions. EMBO J 15:2452–2467
14. Cho HS, Mason K, Ramyar KX, Stanley AM, Gabelli SB, Denney DW Jr, Leahy DJ (2003) Structure of the extracellular region of HER2 alone and in complex with the Herceptin Fab. Nature 421:756–760
15. Karunagaran D, Tzahar E, Beerli RR, Chen X, Graus-Porta D, Ratzkin BJ, Seger R, Hynes NE, Yarden Y (1996) ErbB-2 is a common auxiliary subunit of NDF and EGF receptors: implications for breast cancer. EMBO J 15:254–264

16. Balana ME, Labriola L, Salatino M, Movsichoff F, Peters G, Charreau EH, Elizalde PV (2001) Activation of ErbB-2 via a hierarchical interaction between ErbB-2 and type I insulin-like growth factor receptor in mammary tumor cells. Oncogene 20:34–47
17. Liu D, Aguirre Ghiso J, Estrada Y, Ossowski L (2002) EGFR is a transducer of the urokinase receptor initiated signal that is required for in vivo growth of a human carcinoma. Cancer Cell 1:445–457
18. Brantley-Sieders DM, Zhuang G, Hicks D, Fang WB, Hwang Y, Cates JM, Coffman K, Jackson D, Bruckheimer E, Muraoka-Cook RS et al (2008) The receptor tyrosine kinase EphA2 promotes mammary adenocarcinoma tumorigenesis and metastatic progression in mice by amplifying ErbB2 signaling. J Clin Invest 118:64–78
19. Zhang X, Gureasko J, Shen K, Cole PA, Kuriyan J (2006) An allosteric mechanism for activation of the kinase domain of epidermal growth factor receptor. Cell 125:1137–1149
20. Pawson T (2004) Specificity in signal transduction: from phosphotyrosine-SH2 domain interactions to complex cellular systems. Cell 116:191–203
21. Jones RB, Gordus A, Krall JA, MacBeath G (2006) A quantitative protein interaction network for the ErbB receptors using protein microarrays. Nature 439:168–174
22. Chen P, Gupta K, Wells A (1994) Cell movement elicited by epidermal growth factor receptor requires kinase and autophosphorylation but is separable from mitogenesis. J Cell Biol 124:547–555
23. Ursini-Siegel J, Schade B, Cardiff RD, Muller WJ (2007) Insights from transgenic mouse models of ERBB2-induced breast cancer. Nat Rev Cancer 7:389–397
24. Amit I, Citri A, Shay T, Lu Y, Katz M, Zhang F, Tarcic G, Siwak D, Lahad J, Jacob-Hirsch J et al (2007) A module of negative feedback regulators defines growth factor signaling. Nat Genet 39:503–512
25. Nagashima T, Shimodaira H, Ide K, Nakakuki T, Tani Y, Takahashi K, Yumoto N, Hatakeyama M (2007) Quantitative transcriptional control of ErbB receptor signaling undergoes graded to biphasic response for cell differentiation. J Biol Chem 282:4045–4056
26. Xie Y, Hung MC (1994) Nuclear localization of p185neu tyrosine kinase and its association with transcriptional transactivation. Biochem Biophys Res Commun 203:1589–1598
27. Lin SY, Makino K, Xia W, Matin A, Wen Y, Kwong KY, Bourguignon L, Hung MC (2001) Nuclear localization of EGF receptor and its potential new role as a transcription factor. Nat Cell Biol 3:802–808
28. Ni CY, Murphy MP, Golde TE, Carpenter G (2001) gamma -Secretase cleavage and nuclear localization of ErbB-4 receptor tyrosine kinase. Science 294:2179–2181
29. Offterdinger M, Schofer C, Weipoltshammer K, Grunt TW (2002) c-erbB-3: a nuclear protein in mammary epithelial cells. J Cell Biol 157:929–939
30. Wang SC, Lien HC, Xia W, Chen IF, Lo HW, Wang Z, Ali-Seyed M, Lee DF, Bartholomeusz G, Ou-Yang F et al (2004) Binding at and transactivation of the COX-2 promoter by nuclear tyrosine kinase receptor ErbB-2. Cancer Cell 6:251–261
31. Bao J, Lin H, Ouyang Y, Lei D, Osman A, Kim TW, Mei L, Dai P, Ohlemiller KK, Ambron RT (2004) Activity-dependent transcription regulation of PSD-95 by neuregulin-1 and Eos. Nat Neurosci 7:1250–1258
32. Scaltriti M, Rojo F, Ocana A, Anido J, Guzman M, Cortes J, Di Cosimo S, Matias-Guiu X, Ramon y Cajal S, Arribas J et al (2007) Expression of p95HER2, a truncated form of the HER2 receptor, and response to anti-HER2 therapies in breast cancer. J Natl Cancer Inst 99:628–638
33. Grasl-Kraupp B, Schausberger E, Hufnagl K, Gerner C, Low-Baselli A, Rossmanith W, Parzefall W, Schulte-Hermann R (2002) A novel mechanism for mitogenic signaling via pro-transforming growth factor alpha within hepatocyte nuclei. Hepatology 35:1372–1380
34. Lo HW, Xia W, Wei Y, Ali-Seyed M, Huang SF, Hung MC (2005) Novel prognostic value of nuclear epidermal growth factor receptor in breast cancer. Cancer Res 65:338–348
35. Wang SC, Nakajima Y, Yu YL, Xia W, Chen CT, Yang CC, McIntush EW, Li LY, Hawke DH, Kobayashi R et al (2006) Tyrosine phosphorylation controls PCNA function through protein stability. Nat Cell Biol 8:1359–1368

36. Hollmen M, Maatta JA, Bald L, Sliwkowski MX, Elenius K (2009) Suppression of breast cancer cell growth by a monoclonal antibody targeting cleavable ErbB4 isoforms. Oncogene 28:1309–1319
37. Kim HP, Yoon YK, Kim JW, Han SW, Hur HS, Park J, Lee JH, Oh DY, Im SA, Bang YJ et al (2009) Lapatinib, a dual EGFR and HER2 tyrosine kinase inhibitor, downregulates thymidylate synthase by inhibiting the nuclear translocation of EGFR and HER2. PLoS ONE 4: e5933
38. Geyer CE, Forster J, Lindquist D, Chan S, Romieu CG, Pienkowski T, Jagiello-Gruszfeld A, Crown J, Chan A, Kaufman B et al (2006) Lapatinib plus capecitabine for HER2-positive advanced breast cancer. N Engl J Med 355:2733–2743
39. Stelling J, Sauer U, Szallasi Z, Doyle FJ 3rd, Doyle J (2004) Robustness of cellular functions. Cell 118:675–685
40. Kirschner M, Gerhart J (1998) Evolvability. Proc Natl Acad Sci USA 95:8420–8427
41. Weinstein IB (2002) Cancer. Addiction to oncogenes–the Achilles heal of cancer. Science 297:63–64
42. Luo J, Solimini NL, Elledge SJ (2009) Principles of cancer therapy: oncogene and non-oncogene addiction. Cell 136:823–837
43. Mahalingam D, Swords R, Carew JS, Nawrocki ST, Bhalla K, Giles FJ (2009) Targeting HSP90 for cancer therapy. Br J Cancer 100:1523–1529
44. Modi S, Sugarman S, Stopeck A, Linden H, Ma W, Kersey K, Johnson RG, Rosen N, Hannah AL, Hudis CA (2008) Phase II trial of the Hsp90 inhibitor tanespimycin (Tan) + trastuzumab (T) in patients (pts) with HER2-positive metastatic breast cancer (MBC). J Clin Oncol 26: abstract 1027
45. Modi S, Miller K, Rosen LS, Schneider B, Chap L, Zhong Z, Kersey K, Hannah AL, Hudis C (2008) Alvespimycin (KOS-1022) and trastuzumab (T): activity in HER2+ metastatic breast cancer (MBC). ASCO 2007 Breast Cancer Symposium: abstract 165
46. Beliakoff J, Bagatell R, Paine-Murrieta G, Taylor CW, Lykkesfeldt AE, Whitesell L (2003) Hormone-refractory breast cancer remains sensitive to the antitumor activity of heat shock protein 90 inhibitors. Clin Cancer Res 9:4961–4971
47. Junttila TT, Akita RW, Parsons K, Fields C, Lewis Phillips GD, Friedman LS, Sampath D, Sliwkowski MX (2009) Ligand-independent HER2/HER3/PI3K complex is disrupted by trastuzumab and is effectively inhibited by the PI3K inhibitor GDC-0941. Cancer Cell 15:429–440
48. Agus DB, Akita RW, Fox WD, Lewis GD, Higgins B, Pisacane PI, Lofgren JA, Tindell C, Evans DP, Maiese K et al (2002) Targeting ligand-activated ErbB2 signaling inhibits breast and prostate tumor growth. Cancer Cell 2:127–137
49. Cortés J, Baselga J, Petrella T, Gelmon K, Fumoleau P, Verma S, Pivot XB, Ross G, Szado T, Gianni L (2009) Pertuzumab monotherapy following trastuzumab-based treatment: Activity and tolerability in patients with advanced HER2- positive breast cancer. J Clin Oncol 27: abstract 1022
50. Kholodenko BN (2006) Cell-signalling dynamics in time and space. Nat Rev Mol Cell Biol 7:165–176
51. Peschard P, Fournier TM, Lamorte L, Naujokas MA, Band H, Langdon WY, Park M (2001) Mutation of the c-Cbl TKB domain binding site on the Met receptor tyrosine kinase converts it into a transforming protein. Mol Cell 8:995–1004
52. Sergina NV, Rausch M, Wang D, Blair J, Hann B, Shokat KM, Moasser MM (2007) Escape from HER-family tyrosine kinase inhibitor therapy by the kinase-inactive HER3. Nature 445:437–441
53. Sassone-Corsi P, Sisson JC, Verma IM (1988) Transcriptional autoregulation of the proto-oncogene fos. Nature 334:314–319
54. Gur G, Rubin C, Katz M, Amit I, Citri A, Nilsson J, Amariglio N, Henriksson R, Rechavi G, Hedman H et al (2004) LRIG1 restricts growth factor signaling by enhancing receptor ubiquitylation and degradation. EMBO J 23:3270–3281

55. Miller JK, Shattuck DL, Ingalla EQ, Yen L, Borowsky AD, Young LJ, Cardiff RD, Carraway KL 3rd, Sweeney C (2008) Suppression of the negative regulator LRIG1 contributes to ErbB2 overexpression in breast cancer. Cancer Res 68:8286–8294
56. Zhang X, Pickin KA, Bose R, Jura N, Cole PA, Kuriyan J (2007) Inhibition of the EGF receptor by binding of MIG6 to an activating kinase domain interface. Nature 450:741–744
57. Anastasi S, Sala G, Huiping C, Caprini E, Russo G, Iacovelli S, Lucini F, Ingvarsson S, Segatto O (2005) Loss of RALT/MIG-6 expression in ERBB2-amplified breast carcinomas enhances ErbB-2 oncogenic potency and favors resistance to Herceptin. Oncogene 24:4540–4548
58. Kim HJ, Taylor LJ, Bar-Sagi D (2007) Spatial regulation of EGFR signaling by Sprouty2. Curr Biol 17:455–461
59. Rubin C, Zwang Y, Vaisman N, Ron D, Yarden Y (2005) Phosphorylation of carboxyl-terminal tyrosines modulates the specificity of Sprouty-2 inhibition of different signaling pathways. J Biol Chem 280:9735–9744
60. Hanafusa H, Torii S, Yasunaga T, Nishida E (2002) Sprouty1 and Sprouty2 provide a control mechanism for the Ras/MAPK signalling pathway. Nat Cell Biol 4:850–858
61. Lo TL, Yusoff P, Fong CW, Guo K, McCaw BJ, Phillips WA, Yang H, Wong ES, Leong HF, Zeng Q et al (2004) The ras/mitogen-activated protein kinase pathway inhibitor and likely tumor suppressor proteins, sprouty 1 and sprouty 2 are deregulated in breast cancer. Cancer Res 64:6127–6136
62. Croce CM (2009) Causes and consequences of microRNA dysregulation in cancer. Nat Rev Genet 10:704–714
63. Yuste L, Montero JC, Esparis-Ogando A, Pandiella A (2005) Activation of ErbB2 by overexpression or by transmembrane neuregulin results in differential signaling and sensitivity to herceptin. Cancer Res 65:6801–6810
64. Moody SE, Sarkisian CJ, Hahn KT, Gunther EJ, Pickup S, Dugan KD, Innocent N, Cardiff RD, Schnall MD, Chodosh LA (2002) Conditional activation of Neu in the mammary epithelium of transgenic mice results in reversible pulmonary metastasis. Cancer Cell 2:451–461
65. Slamon DJ, Clark GM, Wong SG, Levin WJ, Ullrich A, McGuire WL (1987) Human breast cancer: correlation of relapse and survival with amplification of the HER-2/neu oncogene. Science 235:177–182
66. Muthuswamy SK, Li D, Lelievre S, Bissell MJ, Brugge JS (2001) ErbB2, but not ErbB1, reinitiates proliferation and induces luminal repopulation in epithelial acini. Nat Cell Biol 3:785–792
67. Zhan L, Xiang B, Muthuswamy SK (2006) Controlled activation of ErbB1/ErbB2 heterodimers promote invasion of three-dimensional organized epithelia in an ErbB1-dependent manner: implications for progression of ErbB2-overexpressing tumors. Cancer Res 66:5201–5208
68. Reginato MJ, Mills KR, Paulus JK, Lynch DK, Sgroi DC, Debnath J, Muthuswamy SK, Brugge JS (2003) Integrins and EGFR coordinately regulate the pro-apoptotic protein Bim to prevent anoikis. Nat Cell Biol 5:733–740
69. Seton-Rogers SE, Lu Y, Hines LM, Koundinya M, LaBaer J, Muthuswamy SK, Brugge JS (2004) Cooperation of the ErbB2 receptor and transforming growth factor beta in induction of migration and invasion in mammary epithelial cells. Proc Natl Acad Sci USA 101:1257–1262
70. Lu J, Guo H, Treekitkarnmongkol W, Li P, Zhang J, Shi B, Ling C, Zhou X, Chen T, Chiao PJ et al (2009) 14-3-3zeta Cooperates with ErbB2 to promote ductal carcinoma in situ progression to invasive breast cancer by inducing epithelial-mesenchymal transition. Cancer Cell 16:195–207
71. van de Vijver M, van de Bersselaar R, Devilee P, Cornelisse C, Peterse J, Nusse R (1987) Amplification of the neu (c-erbB-2) oncogene in human mammmary tumors is relatively frequent and is often accompanied by amplification of the linked c-erbA oncogene. Mol Cell Biol 7:2019–2023

72. Reinholz MM, Bruzek AK, Visscher DW, Lingle WL, Schroeder MJ, Perez EA, Jenkins RB (2009) Breast cancer and aneusomy 17: implications for carcinogenesis and therapeutic response. Lancet Oncol 10:267–277
73. Menendez JA, Lupu R (2007) Fatty acid synthase and the lipogenic phenotype in cancer pathogenesis. Nat Rev Cancer 7:763–777
74. Kraus MH, Popescu NC, Amsbaugh SC, King CR (1987) Overexpression of the EGF receptor-related proto-oncogene erbB-2 in human mammary tumor cell lines by different molecular mechanisms. EMBO J 6:605–610
75. Zuo T, Wang L, Morrison C, Chang X, Zhang H, Li W, Liu Y, Wang Y, Liu X, Chan MW et al (2007) FOXP3 is an X-linked breast cancer suppressor gene and an important repressor of the HER-2/ErbB2 oncogene. Cell 129:1275–1286
76. Xing X, Wang SC, Xia W, Zou Y, Shao R, Kwong KY, Yu Z, Zhang S, Miller S, Huang L et al (2000) The ets protein PEA3 suppresses HER-2/neu overexpression and inhibits tumorigenesis. Nat Med 6:189–195
77. Anido J, Scaltriti M, Bech Serra JJ, Santiago Josefat B, Todo FR, Baselga J, Arribas J (2006) Biosynthesis of tumorigenic HER2 C-terminal fragments by alternative initiation of translation. EMBO J 25:3234–3244
78. Codony-Servat J, Albanell J, Lopez-Talavera JC, Arribas J, Baselga J (1999) Cleavage of the HER2 ectodomain is a pervanadate-activable process that is inhibited by the tissue inhibitor of metalloproteases-1 in breast cancer cells. Cancer Res 59:1196–1201
79. Pedersen K, Angelini PD, Laos S, Bach-Faig A, Cunningham MP, Ferrer-Ramon C, Luque-Garcia A, Garcia-Castillo J, Parra-Palau JL, Scaltriti M et al (2009) A naturally occurring HER2 carboxy-terminal fragment promotes mammary tumor growth and metastasis. Mol Cell Biol 29:3319–3331
80. Xia W, Liu LH, Ho P, Spector NL (2004) Truncated ErbB2 receptor (p95ErbB2) is regulated by heregulin through heterodimer formation with ErbB3 yet remains sensitive to the dual EGFR/ErbB2 kinase inhibitor GW572016. Oncogene 23:646–653
81. Saez R, Molina MA, Ramsey EE, Rojo F, Keenan EJ, Albanell J, Lluch A, Garcia-Conde J, Baselga J, Clinton GM (2006) p95HER-2 predicts worse outcome in patients with HER-2-positive breast cancer. Clin Cancer Res 12:424–431
82. Hudelist G, Kostler WJ, Attems J, Czerwenka K, Muller R, Manavi M, Steger GG, Kubista E, Zielinski CC, Singer CF (2003) Her-2/neu-triggered intracellular tyrosine kinase activation: in vivo relevance of ligand-independent activation mechanisms and impact upon the efficacy of trastuzumab-based treatment. Br J Cancer 89:983–991
83. Scaltriti M, Verma C, Guzman M, Jimenez J, Parra JL, Pedersen K, Smith DJ, Landolfi S, Ramon y Cajal S, Arribas J et al (2009) Lapatinib, a HER2 tyrosine kinase inhibitor, induces stabilization and accumulation of HER2 and potentiates trastuzumab-dependent cell cytotoxicity. Oncogene 28:803–814
84. Pegram MD, Lipton A, Hayes DF, Weber BL, Baselga JM, Tripathy D, Baly D, Baughman SA, Twaddell T, Glaspy JA et al (1998) Phase II study of receptor-enhanced chemosensitivity using recombinant humanized anti-p185HER2/neu monoclonal antibody plus cisplatin in patients with HER2/neu-overexpressing metastatic breast cancer refractory to chemotherapy treatment. J Clin Oncol 16:2659–2671
85. Brodowicz T, Wiltschke C, Budinsky AC, Krainer M, Steger GG, Zielinski CC (1997) Soluble HER-2/neu neutralizes biologic effects of anti-HER-2/neu antibody on breast cancer cells in vitro. Int J Cancer 73:875–879
86. Molina MA, Codony-Servat J, Albanell J, Rojo F, Arribas J, Baselga J (2001) Trastuzumab (herceptin), a humanized anti-Her2 receptor monoclonal antibody, inhibits basal and activated Her2 ectodomain cleavage in breast cancer cells. Cancer Res 61:4744–4749
87. Ali SM, Carney WP, Esteva FJ, Fornier M, Harris L, Kostler WJ, Lotz JP, Luftner D, Pichon MF, Lipton A (2008) Serum HER-2/neu and relative resistance to trastuzumab-based therapy in patients with metastatic breast cancer. Cancer 113:1294–1301
88. Kostler WJ, Schwab B, Singer CF, Neumann R, Rucklinger E, Brodowicz T, Tomek S, Niedermayr M, Hejna M, Steger GG et al (2004) Monitoring of serum Her-2/neu predicts

response and progression-free survival to trastuzumab-based treatment in patients with metastatic breast cancer. Clin Cancer Res 10:1618–1624
89. Siegel PM, Ryan ED, Cardiff RD, Muller WJ (1999) Elevated expression of activated forms of Neu/ErbB-2 and ErbB-3 are involved in the induction of mammary tumors in transgenic mice: implications for human breast cancer. EMBO J 18:2149–2164
90. Nagata Y, Lan KH, Zhou X, Tan M, Esteva FJ, Sahin AA, Klos KS, Li P, Monia BP, Nguyen NT et al (2004) PTEN activation contributes to tumor inhibition by trastuzumab, and loss of PTEN predicts trastuzumab resistance in patients. Cancer Cell 6:117–127
91. Mitra D, Brumlik MJ, Okamgba SU, Zhu Y, Duplessis TT, Parvani JG, Lesko SM, Brogi E, Jones FE (2009) An oncogenic isoform of HER2 associated with locally disseminated breast cancer and trastuzumab resistance. Mol Cancer Ther 8(8):2152–2162
92. Kwong KY, Hung MC (1998) A novel splice variant of HER2 with increased transformation activity. Mol Carcinog 23:62–68
93. Moscatello DK, Holgado-Madruga M, Godwin AK, Ramirez G, Gunn G, Zoltick PW, Biegel JA, Hayes RL, Wong AJ (1995) Frequent expression of a mutant epidermal growth factor receptor in multiple human tumors. Cancer Res 55:5536–5539
94. Nieto Y, Nawaz F, Jones RB, Shpall EJ, Nawaz S (2007) Prognostic significance of overexpression and phosphorylation of epidermal growth factor receptor (EGFR) and the presence of truncated EGFRvIII in locoregionally advanced breast cancer. J Clin Oncol 25:4405–4413
95. Moscatello DK, Holgado-Madruga M, Emlet DR, Montgomery RB, Wong AJ (1998) Constitutive activation of phosphatidylinositol 3-kinase by a naturally occurring mutant epidermal growth factor receptor. J Biol Chem 273:200–206
96. Fan QW, Knight ZA, Goldenberg DD, Yu W, Mostov KE, Stokoe D, Shokat KM, Weiss WA (2006) A dual PI3 kinase/mTOR inhibitor reveals emergent efficacy in glioma. Cancer Cell 9:341–349
97. Garrett TP, Burgess AW, Gan HK, Luwor RB, Cartwright G, Walker F, Orchard SG, Clayton AH, Nice EC, Rothacker J et al (2009) Antibodies specifically targeting a locally misfolded region of tumor associated EGFR. Proc Natl Acad Sci USA 106:5082–5087
98. Borrell-Pages M, Rojo F, Albanell J, Baselga J, Arribas J (2003) TACE is required for the activation of the EGFR by TGF-alpha in tumors. EMBO J 22:1114–1124
99. Marcotte R, Muller WJ (2008) Signal transduction in transgenic mouse models of human breast cancer–implications for human breast cancer. J Mammary Gland Biol Neoplasia 13:323–335
100. Earp HS, Austin KS, Blaisdell J, Rubin RA, Nelson KG, Lee LW, Grisham JW (1986) Epidermal growth factor (EGF) stimulates EGF receptor synthesis. J Biol Chem 261: 4777–4780
101. Schroeder JA, Troyer KL, Lee DC (2000) Cooperative induction of mammary tumorigenesis by TGFalpha and Wnts. Oncogene 19:3193–3199
102. Wyckoff J, Wang W, Lin EY, Wang Y, Pixley F, Stanley ER, Graf T, Pollard JW, Segall J, Condeelis J (2004) A paracrine loop between tumor cells and macrophages is required for tumor cell migration in mammary tumors. Cancer Res 64:7022–7029
103. Lu X, Wang Q, Hu G, Van Poznak C, Fleisher M, Reiss M, Massague J, Kang Y (2009) ADAMTS1 and MMP1 proteolytically engage EGF-like ligands in an osteolytic signaling cascade for bone metastasis. Genes Dev 23:1882–1894
104. Tagliabue E, Agresti R, Carcangiu ML, Ghirelli C, Morelli D, Campiglio M, Martel M, Giovanazzi R, Greco M, Balsari A et al (2003) Role of HER2 in wound-induced breast carcinoma proliferation. Lancet 362:527–533
105. Singer CF, Hudelist G, Fuchs EM, Kostler W, Fink-Retter A, Gschwantler-Kaulich D, Gnant M, Lamm W, Rudas M, Czerwenka K et al (2009) Incomplete surgical resection of ductal carcinomas in situ results in activation of ERBB2 in residual breast cancer cells. Endocr Relat Cancer 16:73–83
106. Motoyama AB, Hynes NE, Lane HA (2002) The efficacy of ErbB receptor-targeted anticancer therapeutics is influenced by the availability of epidermal growth factor-related peptides. Cancer Res 62:3151–3158

107. Hayes NV, Gullick WJ (2008) The neuregulin family of genes and their multiple splice variants in breast cancer. J Mammary Gland Biol Neoplasia 13:205–214
108. Biscardi JS, Ishizawar RC, Silva CM, Parsons SJ (2000) Tyrosine kinase signalling in breast cancer: epidermal growth factor receptor and c-Src interactions in breast cancer. Breast Cancer Res 2:203–210
109. Guo W, Pylayeva Y, Pepe A, Yoshioka T, Muller WJ, Inghirami G, Giancotti FG (2006) Beta 4 integrin amplifies ErbB2 signaling to promote mammary tumorigenesis. Cell 126:489–502
110. Mueller KL, Hunter LA, Ethier SP, Boerner JL (2008) Met and c-Src cooperate to compensate for loss of epidermal growth factor receptor kinase activity in breast cancer cells. Cancer Res 68:3314–3322
111. Chaturvedi D, Gao X, Cohen MS, Taunton J, Patel TB (2009) Rapamycin induces transactivation of the EGFR and increases cell survival. Oncogene 28:1187–1196
112. Kim H, Chan R, Dankort DL, Zuo D, Najoukas M, Park M, Muller WJ (2005) The c-Src tyrosine kinase associates with the catalytic domain of ErbB-2: implications for ErbB-2 mediated signaling and transformation. Oncogene 24:7599–7607
113. Muthuswamy SK, Siegel PM, Dankort DL, Webster MA, Muller WJ (1994) Mammary tumors expressing the neu proto-oncogene possess elevated c-Src tyrosine kinase activity. Mol Cell Biol 14:735–743
114. Ishizawar RC, Miyake T, Parsons SJ (2007) c-Src modulates ErbB2 and ErbB3 heterocomplex formation and function. Oncogene 26:3503–3510
115. Yeatman TJ (2004) A renaissance for SRC. Nat Rev Cancer 4:470–480
116. Migliaccio A, Piccolo D, Castoria G, Di Domenico M, Bilancio A, Lombardi M, Gong W, Beato M, Auricchio F (1998) Activation of the Src/p21ras/Erk pathway by progesterone receptor via cross-talk with estrogen receptor. EMBO J 17:2008–2018
117. Bai T, Luoh SW (2008) GRB-7 facilitates HER-2/Neu-mediated signal transduction and tumor formation. Carcinogenesis 29:473–479
118. Stein D, Wu J, Fuqua SA, Roonprapunt C, Yajnik V, D'Eustachio P, Moskow JJ, Buchberg AM, Osborne CK, Margolis B (1994) The SH2 domain protein GRB-7 is co-amplified, overexpressed and in a tight complex with HER2 in breast cancer. EMBO J 13:1331–1340
119. Arteaga CL, Johnson MD, Todderud G, Coffey RJ, Carpenter G, Page DL (1991) Elevated content of the tyrosine kinase substrate phospholipase C-gamma 1 in primary human breast carcinomas. Proc Natl Acad Sci USA 88:10435–10439
120. Lowenstein EJ, Daly RJ, Batzer AG, Li W, Margolis B, Lammers R, Ullrich A, Skolnik EY, Bar-Sagi D, Schlessinger J (1992) The SH2 and SH3 domain-containing protein GRB2 links receptor tyrosine kinases to ras signaling. Cell 70:431–442
121. Daly RJ, Binder MD, Sutherland RL (1994) Overexpression of the Grb2 gene in human breast cancer cell lines. Oncogene 9:2723–2727
122. Bentires-Alj M, Gil SG, Chan R, Wang ZC, Wang Y, Imanaka N, Harris LN, Richardson A, Neel BG, Gu H (2006) A role for the scaffolding adapter GAB2 in breast cancer. Nat Med 12:114–121
123. Bromberg JF, Wrzeszczynska MH, Devgan G, Zhao Y, Pestell RG, Albanese C, Darnell JE Jr (1999) Stat3 as an oncogene. Cell 98:295–303
124. Ranger JJ, Levy DE, Shahalizadeh S, Hallett M, Muller WJ (2009) Identification of a Stat3-dependent transcription regulatory network involved in metastatic progression. Cancer Res 69:6823–6830
125. Bellacosa A, de Feo D, Godwin AK, Bell DW, Cheng JQ, Altomare DA, Wan M, Dubeau L, Scambia G, Masciullo V et al (1995) Molecular alterations of the AKT2 oncogene in ovarian and breast carcinomas. Int J Cancer 64:280–285
126. Xiang B, Chatti K, Qiu H, Lakshmi B, Krasnitz A, Hicks J, Yu M, Miller WT, Muthuswamy SK (2008) Brk is coamplified with ErbB2 to promote proliferation in breast cancer. Proc Natl Acad Sci USA 105:12463–12468
127. Philippar U, Roussos ET, Oser M, Yamaguchi H, Kim HD, Giampieri S, Wang Y, Goswami S, Wyckoff JB, Lauffenburger DA et al (2008) A Mena invasion isoform potentiates EGF-induced carcinoma cell invasion and metastasis. Dev Cell 15:813–828

128. Samuels Y, Wang Z, Bardelli A, Silliman N, Ptak J, Szabo S, Yan H, Gazdar A, Powell SM, Riggins GJ et al (2004) High frequency of mutations of the PIK3CA gene in human cancers. Science 304:554
129. Gustin JP, Karakas B, Weiss MB, Abukhdeir AM, Lauring J, Garay JP, Cosgrove D, Tamaki A, Konishi H, Konishi Y et al (2009) Knockin of mutant PIK3CA activates multiple oncogenic pathways. Proc Natl Acad Sci USA 106:2835–2840
130. Stemke-Hale K, Gonzalez-Angulo AM, Lluch A, Neve RM, Kuo WL, Davies M, Carey M, Hu Z, Guan Y, Sahin A et al (2008) An integrative genomic and proteomic analysis of PIK3CA, PTEN, and AKT mutations in breast cancer. Cancer Res 68:6084–6091
131. Saal LH, Holm K, Maurer M, Memeo L, Su T, Wang X, Yu JS, Malmstrom PO, Mansukhani M, Enoksson J et al (2005) PIK3CA mutations correlate with hormone receptors, node metastasis, and ERBB2, and are mutually exclusive with PTEN loss in human breast carcinoma. Cancer Res 65:2554–2559
132. Maurer M, Su T, Saal LH, Koujak S, Hopkins BD, Barkley CR, Wu J, Nandula S, Dutta B, Xie Y et al (2009) 3-Phosphoinositide-dependent kinase 1 potentiates upstream lesions on the phosphatidylinositol 3-kinase pathway in breast carcinoma. Cancer Res 69:6299–6306
133. Tseng PH, Wang YC, Weng SC, Weng JR, Chen CS, Brueggemeier RW, Shapiro CL, Chen CY, Dunn SE, Pollak M (2006) Overcoming trastuzumab resistance in HER2-overexpressing breast cancer cells by using a novel celecoxib-derived phosphoinositide-dependent kinase-1 inhibitor. Mol Pharmacol 70:1534–1541
134. Carpten JD, Faber AL, Horn C, Donoho GP, Briggs SL, Robbins CM, Hostetter G, Boguslawski S, Moses TY, Savage S et al (2007) A transforming mutation in the pleckstrin homology domain of AKT1 in cancer. Nature 448:439–444
135. Liu H, Radisky DC, Nelson CM, Zhang H, Fata JE, Roth RA, Bissell MJ (2006) Mechanism of Akt1 inhibition of breast cancer cell invasion reveals a protumorigenic role for TSC2. Proc Natl Acad Sci USA 103:4134–4139
136. Hutchinson JN, Jin J, Cardiff RD, Woodgett JR, Muller WJ (2004) Activation of Akt-1 (PKB-alpha) can accelerate ErbB-2-mediated mammary tumorigenesis but suppresses tumor invasion. Cancer Res 64:3171–3178
137. Irie HY, Pearline RV, Grueneberg D, Hsia M, Ravichandran P, Kothari N, Natesan S, Brugge JS (2005) Distinct roles of Akt1 and Akt2 in regulating cell migration and epithelial-mesenchymal transition. J Cell Biol 171:1023–1034
138. Mosesson Y, Mills GB, Yarden Y (2008) Derailed endocytosis: an emerging feature of cancer. Nat Rev Cancer 8:835–850
139. Zwang Y, Yarden Y (2009) Systems biology of growth factor-induced receptor endocytosis. Traffic 10:349–363
140. Levkowitz G, Waterman H, Zamir E, Kam Z, Oved S, Langdon WY, Beguinot L, Geiger B, Yarden Y (1998) c-Cbl/Sli-1 regulates endocytic sorting and ubiquitination of the epidermal growth factor receptor. Genes Dev 12:3663–3674
141. Wang Y, Du D, Fang L, Yang G, Zhang C, Zeng R, Ullrich A, Lottspeich F, Chen Z (2006) Tyrosine phosphorylated Par3 regulates epithelial tight junction assembly promoted by EGFR signaling. EMBO J 25:5058–5070
142. Aranda V, Haire T, Nolan ME, Calarco JP, Rosenberg AZ, Fawcett JP, Pawson T, Muthuswamy SK (2006) Par6-aPKC uncouples ErbB2 induced disruption of polarized epithelial organization from proliferation control. Nat Cell Biol 8:1235–1245
143. Morishige M, Hashimoto S, Ogawa E, Toda Y, Kotani H, Hirose M, Wei S, Hashimoto A, Yamada A, Yano H et al (2008) GEP100 links epidermal growth factor receptor signalling to Arf6 activation to induce breast cancer invasion. Nat Cell Biol 10:85–92
144. Sorkin A, Von Zastrow M (2002) Signal transduction and endocytosis: close encounters of many kinds. Nat Rev Mol Cell Biol 3:600–614
145. French AR, Sudlow GP, Wiley HS, Lauffenburger DA (1994) Postendocytic trafficking of epidermal growth factor-receptor complexes is mediated through saturable and specific endosomal interactions. J Biol Chem 269:15749–15755

146. Wilde A, Beattie EC, Lem L, Riethof DA, Liu SH, Mobley WC, Soriano P, Brodsky FM (1999) EGF receptor signaling stimulates SRC kinase phosphorylation of clathrin, influencing clathrin redistribution and EGF uptake. Cell 96:677–687
147. Bao J, Gur G, Yarden Y (2003) Src promotes destruction of c-Cbl: implications for oncogenic synergy between Src and growth factor receptors. Proc Natl Acad Sci USA 100:2438–2443
148. Thien CB, Langdon WY (2001) Cbl: many adaptations to regulate protein tyrosine kinases. Nat Rev Mol Cell Biol 2:294–307
149. Murphy MA, Schnall RG, Venter DJ, Barnett L, Bertoncello I, Thien CB, Langdon WY, Bowtell DD (1998) Tissue hyperplasia and enhanced T-cell signalling via ZAP-70 in c-Cbl-deficient mice. Mol Cell Biol 18:4872–4882
150. Kochupurakkal BS, Harari D, Di-Segni A, Maik-Rachline G, Lyass L, Gur G, Kerber G, Citri A, Lavi S, Eilam R et al (2005) Epigen, the last ligand of ErbB receptors, reveals intricate relationships between affinity and mitogenicity. J Biol Chem 280:8503–8512
151. French AR, Tadaki DK, Niyogi SK, Lauffenburger DA (1995) Intracellular trafficking of epidermal growth factor family ligands is directly influenced by the pH sensitivity of the receptor/ligand interaction. J Biol Chem 270:4334–4340
152. Grandal MV, Zandi R, Pedersen MW, Willumsen BM, van Deurs B, Poulsen HS (2007) EGFRvIII escapes down-regulation due to impaired internalization and sorting to lysosomes. Carcinogenesis 28:1408–1417
153. Offterdinger M, Bastiaens PI (2008) Prolonged EGFR Signaling by ERBB2-Mediated Sequestration at the Plasma Membrane. Traffic 9:147–155
154. Baulida J, Kraus MH, Alimandi M, Di Fiore PP, Carpenter G (1996) All ErbB receptors other than the epidermal growth factor receptor are endocytosis impaired. J Biol Chem 271:5251–5257
155. Lenferink AE, Pinkas-Kramarski R, van de Poll ML, van Vugt MJ, Klapper LN, Tzahar E, Waterman H, Sela M, van Zoelen EJ, Yarden Y (1998) Differential endocytic routing of homo- and hetero-dimeric ErbB tyrosine kinases confers signaling superiority to receptor heterodimers. EMBO J 17:3385–3397
156. Shelly M, Pinkas-Kramarski R, Guarino BC, Waterman H, Wang LM, Lyass L, Alimandi M, Kuo A, Bacus SS, Pierce JH et al (1998) Epiregulin is a potent pan-ErbB ligand that preferentially activates heterodimeric receptor complexes. J Biol Chem 273:10496–10505
157. Feng Q, Baird D, Peng X, Wang J, Ly T, Guan JL, Cerione RA (2006) Cool-1 functions as an essential regulatory node for EGF receptor- and Src-mediated cell growth. Nat Cell Biol 8:945–956
158. Wu WJ, Tu S, Cerione RA (2003) Activated Cdc42 sequesters c-Cbl and prevents EGF receptor degradation. Cell 114:715–725
159. Hui R, Campbell DH, Lee CS, McCaul K, Horsfall DJ, Musgrove EA, Daly RJ, Seshadri R, Sutherland RL (1997) EMS1 amplification can occur independently of CCND1 or INT-2 amplification at 11q13 and may identify different phenotypes in primary breast cancer. Oncogene 15:1617–1623
160. Timpson P, Lynch DK, Schramek D, Walker F, Daly RJ (2005) Cortactin overexpression inhibits ligand-induced down-regulation of the epidermal growth factor receptor. Cancer Res 65:3273–3280
161. Ostman A, Hellberg C, Bohmer FD (2006) Protein-tyrosine phosphatases and cancer. Nat Rev Cancer 6:307–320
162. Liebow C, Reilly C, Serrano M, Schally AV (1989) Somatostatin analogues inhibit growth of pancreatic cancer by stimulating tyrosine phosphatase. Proc Natl Acad Sci USA 86:2003–2007
163. Prasad NK, Tandon M, Badve S, Snyder PW, Nakshatri H (2008) Phosphoinositol phosphatase SHIP2 promotes cancer development and metastasis coupled with alterations in EGF receptor turnover. Carcinogenesis 29:25–34
164. Stambolic V, Suzuki A, de la Pompa JL, Brothers GM, Mirtsos C, Sasaki T, Ruland J, Penninger JM, Siderovski DP, Mak TW (1998) Negative regulation of PKB/Akt-dependent cell survival by the tumor suppressor PTEN. Cell 95:29–39

165. Miller TW, Perez-Torres M, Narasanna A, Guix M, Stal O, Perez-Tenorio G, Gonzalez-Angulo AM, Hennessy BT, Mills GB, Kennedy JP et al (2009) Loss of Phosphatase and Tensin homologue deleted on chromosome 10 engages ErbB3 and insulin-like growth factor-I receptor signaling to promote antiestrogen resistance in breast cancer. Cancer Res 69:4192–4201
166. Yin Y, Shen WH (2008) PTEN: a new guardian of the genome. Oncogene 27:5443–5453
167. Lane HA, Beuvink I, Motoyama AB, Daly JM, Neve RM, Hynes NE (2000) ErbB2 potentiates breast tumor proliferation through modulation of p27(Kip1)-Cdk2 complex formation: receptor overexpression does not determine growth dependency. Mol Cell Biol 20:3210–3223
168. Yakes FM, Chinratanalab W, Ritter CA, King W, Seelig S, Arteaga CL (2002) Herceptin-induced inhibition of phosphatidylinositol-3 kinase and Akt Is required for antibody-mediated effects on p27, cyclin D1, and antitumor action. Cancer Res 62:4132–4141
169. Nahta R, Takahashi T, Ueno NT, Hung MC, Esteva FJ (2004) P27(kip1) down-regulation is associated with trastuzumab resistance in breast cancer cells. Cancer Res 64:3981–3986
170. Muraoka RS, Lenferink AE, Law B, Hamilton E, Brantley DM, Roebuck LR, Arteaga CL (2002) ErbB2/Neu-induced, cyclin D1-dependent transformation is accelerated in p27-haploinsufficient mammary epithelial cells but impaired in p27-null cells. Mol Cell Biol 22:2204–2219
171. Bianco R, Shin I, Ritter CA, Yakes FM, Basso A, Rosen N, Tsurutani J, Dennis PA, Mills GB, Arteaga CL (2003) Loss of PTEN/MMAC1/TEP in EGF receptor-expressing tumor cells counteracts the antitumor action of EGFR tyrosine kinase inhibitors. Oncogene 22:2812–2822
172. She QB, Solit D, Basso A, Moasser MM (2003) Resistance to gefitinib in PTEN-null HER-overexpressing tumor cells can be overcome through restoration of PTEN function or pharmacologic modulation of constitutive phosphatidylinositol 3′-kinase/Akt pathway signaling. Clin Cancer Res 9:4340–4346
173. Robinson AG, Turbin D, Thomson T, Yorida E, Ellard S, Bajdik C, Huntsman D, Gelmon K (2006) Molecular predictive factors in patients receiving trastuzumab-based chemotherapy for metastatic disease. Clin Breast Cancer 7:254–261
174. Eichhorn PJ, Gili M, Scaltriti M, Serra V, Guzman M, Nijkamp W, Beijersbergen RL, Valero V, Seoane J, Bernards R et al (2008) Phosphatidylinositol 3-kinase hyperactivation results in lapatinib resistance that is reversed by the mTOR/phosphatidylinositol 3-kinase inhibitor NVP-BEZ235. Cancer Res 68:9221–9230
175. Johnston S, Trudeau M, Kaufman B, Boussen H, Blackwell K, LoRusso P, Lombardi DP, Ben Ahmed S, Citrin DL, DeSilvio ML et al (2008) Phase II study of predictive biomarker profiles for response targeting human epidermal growth factor receptor 2 (HER-2) in advanced inflammatory breast cancer with lapatinib monotherapy. J Clin Oncol 26:1066–1072
176. Xia W, Husain I, Liu L, Bacus S, Saini S, Spohn J, Pry K, Westlund R, Stein SH, Spector NL (2007) Lapatinib antitumor activity is not dependent upon phosphatase and tensin homologue deleted on chromosome 10 in ErbB2-overexpressing breast cancers. Cancer Res 67:1170–1175
177. Faratian D, Goltsov A, Lebedeva G, Sorokin A, Moodie S, Mullen P, Kay C, Um IH, Langdon S, Goryanin I et al (2009) Systems biology reveals new strategies for personalizing cancer medicine and confirms the role of PTEN in resistance to trastuzumab. Cancer Res 69:6713–6720
178. Hornberg JJ, Bruggeman FJ, Westerhoff HV, Lankelma J (2006) Cancer: a Systems Biology disease. Biosystems 83:81–90
179. Um SH, Frigerio F, Watanabe M, Picard F, Joaquin M, Sticker M, Fumagalli S, Allegrini PR, Kozma SC, Auwerx J et al (2004) Absence of S6K1 protects against age- and diet-induced obesity while enhancing insulin sensitivity. Nature 431:200–205
180. Sarbassov DD, Guertin DA, Ali SM, Sabatini DM (2005) Phosphorylation and regulation of Akt/PKB by the rictor-mTOR complex. Science 307:1098–1101

181. Carracedo A, Ma L, Teruya-Feldstein J, Rojo F, Salmena L, Alimonti A, Egia A, Sasaki AT, Thomas G, Kozma SC et al (2008) Inhibition of mTORC1 leads to MAPK pathway activation through a PI3K-dependent feedback loop in human cancer. J Clin Invest 118:3065–3074
182. Guertin DA, Sabatini DM (2007) Defining the role of mTOR in cancer. Cancer Cell 12:9–22
183. Chan S, Scheulen ME, Johnston S, Mross K, Cardoso F, Dittrich C, Eiermann W, Hess D, Morant R, Semiglazov V et al (2005) Phase II study of temsirolimus (CCI-779), a novel inhibitor of mTOR, in heavily pretreated patients with locally advanced or metastatic breast cancer. J Clin Oncol 23:5314–5322
184. O'Reilly KE, Rojo F, She QB, Solit D, Mills GB, Smith D, Lane H, Hofmann F, Hicklin DJ, Ludwig DL et al (2006) mTOR inhibition induces upstream receptor tyrosine kinase signaling and activates Akt. Cancer Res 66:1500–1508
185. Nahta R, Yuan LX, Du Y, Esteva FJ (2007) Lapatinib induces apoptosis in trastuzumab-resistant breast cancer cells: effects on insulin-like growth factor I signaling. Mol Cancer Ther 6:667–674
186. Lu CH, Wyszomierski SL, Tseng LM, Sun MH, Lan KH, Neal CL, Mills GB, Hortobagyi GN, Esteva FJ, Yu D (2007) Preclinical testing of clinically applicable strategies for overcoming trastuzumab resistance caused by PTEN deficiency. Clin Cancer Res 13:5883–5888
187. Wang LH, Chan JL, Li W (2007) Rapamycin together with herceptin significantly increased anti-tumor efficacy compared to either alone in ErbB2 over expressing breast cancer cells. Int J Cancer 121:157–164
188. Berns K, Horlings HM, Hennessy BT, Madiredjo M, Hijmans EM, Beelen K, Linn SC, Gonzalez-Angulo AM, Stemke-Hale K, Hauptmann M et al (2007) A functional genetic approach identifies the PI3K pathway as a major determinant of trastuzumab resistance in breast cancer. Cancer Cell 12:395–402
189. Migliaccio I, Gutierrez M, Wu M, Wong H, Pavlick A, Hilsenbeck SG, Horlings HM, Rimawi M, Berns K, Bernards R et al (2009) PI3 kinase activation and response to trastuzumab or lapatinib in HER-2 overexpressing locally advanced breast cancer (LABC). Cancer Res 69: abstract 34
190. Bianco R, Garofalo S, Rosa R, Damiano V, Gelardi T, Daniele G, Marciano R, Ciardiello F, Tortora G (2008) Inhibition of mTOR pathway by everolimus cooperates with EGFR inhibitors in human tumours sensitive and resistant to anti-EGFR drugs. Br J Cancer 98:923–930
191. Adjei AA, Cohen RB, Franklin W, Morris C, Wilson D, Molina JR, Hanson LJ, Gore L, Chow L, Leong S et al (2008) Phase I pharmacokinetic and pharmacodynamic study of the oral, small-molecule mitogen-activated protein kinase kinase 1/2 inhibitor AZD6244 (ARRY-142886) in patients with advanced cancers. J Clin Oncol 26:2139–2146
192. Mirzoeva OK, Das D, Heiser LM, Bhattacharya S, Siwak D, Gendelman R, Bayani N, Wang NJ, Neve RM, Guan Y et al (2009) Basal subtype and MAPK/ERK kinase (MEK)-phosphoinositide 3-kinase feedback signaling determine susceptibility of breast cancer cells to MEK inhibition. Cancer Res 69:565–572
193. Di Nicolantonio F, Martini M, Molinari F, Sartore-Bianchi A, Arena S, Saletti P, De Dosso S, Mazzucchelli L, Frattini M, Siena S et al (2008) Wild-type BRAF is required for response to panitumumab or cetuximab in metastatic colorectal cancer. J Clin Oncol 26:5705–5712
194. Bild AH, Yao G, Chang JT, Wang Q, Potti A, Chasse D, Joshi MB, Harpole D, Lancaster JM, Berchuck A et al (2006) Oncogenic pathway signatures in human cancers as a guide to targeted therapies. Nature 439:353–357
195. Chang JT, Carvalho C, Mori S, Bild AH, Gatza ML, Wang Q, Lucas JE, Potti A, Febbo PG, West M et al (2009) A genomic strategy to elucidate modules of oncogenic pathway signaling networks. Mol Cell 34:104–114
196. Wiley HS, Cunningham DD (1981) A steady state model for analyzing the cellular binding, internalization and degradation of polypeptide ligands. Cell 25:433–440
197. Kholodenko BN, Demin OV, Moehren G, Hoek JB (1999) Quantification of short term signaling by the epidermal growth factor receptor. J Biol Chem 274:30169–30181

Trastuzumab as Adjuvant Treatment for Early Stage HER-2-positive Breast Cancer

Rupert Bartsch and Guenther G. Steger

Abstract Her-2-positive breast cancers are associated with higher recurrence rates and increased mortality. Trastuzumab, a humanised monoclonal antibody targeting the extracellular domain of Her-2, is an important part of palliative first-line therapy. Combination therapy with taxanes improved response rates, progression-free as well as overall survival.

Based on those results, different groups initiated prospective randomised phase III trials evaluating the role of trastuzumab in the adjuvant setting. Again, significantly superior outcomes were observed in terms of recurrence-free and overall survival. Importantly however, a recently presented French trial showed no additional benefit of trastuzumab over conventional chemotherapy alone. As the mentioned adjuvant studies had huge differences in their respective designs, a number of questions remain unanswered; furthermore, those differences may account for disparities in both, efficacy and side effects.

In the neo-adjuvant setting, the addition of trastuzumab to conventional chemotherapy yielded pathologic complete remission rates of up to 60%. Therefore, preoperative therapy regimens of Her-2-positive tumours today should incorporate trastuzumab.

As reported from earlier studies, cardiotoxicity appears to be the most significant side effect of trastuzumab treatment; this apparently is most prominent if the antibody is administered closely to an anthracycline.

In this chapter, current knowledge of the role of trastuzumab in the adjuvant setting is discussed.

G.G. Steger (✉)
Department of Medicine 1 and Cancer Centre, Clinical Division of Oncology, Medical University of Vienna, Waehringer Guertel 18-20, 1090 Vienna, Austria
e-mail: guenther.steger@meduniwien.ac.at

M. Sibilia et al. (eds.), *Drugs for HER-2-positive Breast Cancer*,
Milestones in Drug Therapy, DOI 10.1007/978-3-0346-0094-1_2,

1 Introduction

Breast cancer remains the most prevalent cancer in women in both, developed and developing countries, and holds responsible for almost half a million deaths per year worldwide [1]. The history of targeted therapies for the treatment of breast cancer dates back to surgical oophorectomy in the late nineteenth century [2]. Today, a wide range of anti-hormonal agents and other targeted drugs, including trastuzumab, bevacizumab and lapatinib are available.

In the 1980s, it was established that patients suffering from Her (Human epidermal growth factor receptor)-2 positive tumours had a more aggressive course of disease [3–5]. Furthermore, it was discovered that Her-2 was a transmembrane growth factor receptor, which in conjunction with other members of the epidermal growth factor super-family (EGFR = Her1; Her3, Her4) will activate downstream signalling pathways important for cell growth and survival. Based on those findings, a humanised monoclonal antibody, trastuzumab (rhMab4D5), targeting Her-2 was developed.

1.1 Role of Her-2 in Healthy Tissue

Her-2 plays a number of physiological roles in healthy tissue. Among others, Her-2 signalling regulates cell differentiation, survival and cell repair mechanism [6]. Of note, cardiac myocytes seem to depend strongly on Her-2-activation in response to stress as caused by anthracyclines [7].

1.2 Assessment of Her-2 Status

Given the importance of Her-2 for tumour growth, reliable evaluation of patients' Her-status is paramount. Her-2-positivity is defined as either increased receptor expression or gene amplification. Two different methods are being used worldwide: immunohistochemistry (IHC) and fluorescence in situ hybridisation (FISH). Other options, including chromogenic in situ hybridisation (CISH) [8] or real-time polymerase chain reaction (RT-PCR) [9], are an established alternative to FISH, while gene expression profiles are still largely considered experimental.

Differences were observed between Her-2-testing in high- and low-volume centres [10]. Therefore, it is recommended that Her-2-status should be assessed in specialised institutions [11].

2 Trastuzumab

For 10 years, the use of trastuzumab is firmly established in Her-2-positive advanced breast cancer. The drug has dramatically increased response rate and progression-free survival as well as overall survival.

2.1 *Mechanism of Action*

Trastuzumab is a recombinant monoclonal humanised antibody targeting the extracellular domain of Her-2. Different mechanisms of action were suggested: Inhibition of downstream signalling pathways; internalisation and degradation of Her-2 receptor protein; p27 induction causing cell cycle arrest due to decreased cyclin-dependent kinase 2 (CDK2) activity; inhibition of DNA repair; and antibody-dependent cellular cytotoxicity (ADCC) [12]. In addition, trastuzumab sensitises tumour cells to the cytotoxic effects of conventional chemotherapy [13]. It is still unclear whether trastuzumab actually causes downregulation of Her-2, as some studies have demonstrated that receptor levels remain basically unchanged [12]. On the other hand, lapatinib, a tyrosine-kinase inhibitor of EGFR and Her-2, was observed to actively inhibit Her-2-internalisation, thereby exposing tumour cells to the immunologic effect of trastuzumab [14]. This mechanism may well hold responsible for the synergistic effect of lapatinib and trastuzumab, which has recently been reported in a randomised study [15].

Phase II clinical trials established the activity of trastuzumab as single-agent in Her-2-positive metastatic breast cancer [16, 17]. Based on those proof-of-principle studies, large randomised trials were initiated. Here, the combination of trastuzumab and taxanes was found superior in terms of response, progression-free and overall survival over chemotherapy alone [18, 19]. Accordingly, trastuzumab was approved as first-line treatment for Her-2-positive metastatic breast cancer in combination with taxanes.

2.2 *Mechanisms of Resistance*

Questions concerning mechanisms of resistance to trastuzumab-based therapy remain largely unresolved. Only one third of patients will initially respond to trastuzumab, suggesting de novo (primary) resistance [20]. Even in responders, acquired (secondary) resistance will eventually develop, as the majority of patients will experience disease progression within 1 year of treatment initiation [12].

A number of escape mechanisms were described, and trastuzumab resistance is likely a multifactorial process [12]. Known pathways conferring resistance comprise: Activation of insulin-like growth factor-1 (IGF-1) and its downstream signalling pathways [21]; phosphatase and tensin homologue loss (PTEN) [22]; increased Akt signalling [23, 24]; steric hindrance of trastuzumab binding to Her-2 by cell surface proteins such as mucin-4 (MUC4) [12]; truncated Her-2 receptor (p95 Her-2), a receptor variant without extracellular domain due to alternative splicing [25]; and downregulation of p27 [12].

With alternative Her-2-targeted drugs becoming available (lapatinib, pertuzumab, trastuzumab-DM1, neratinib, ...), the question of specific mechanisms of resistance will gain importance and answers will ultimately help finding the optimal treatment approach for Her-2-positive tumours.

2.3 Combination of Chemotherapy with Trastuzumab in Advanced Breast Cancer

Based on preclinical studies conducted by Pegram et al., cytotoxic agents and trastuzumab were classed either as synergistic, agonistic or antagonistic [13]. Data were derived from cell culture as well as a tumour xenograft model. Based upon those results, special emphasis was put on combinations with taxanes, vinorelbine and platinum compounds (as for those substances a synergistic interaction was hypothesised).

As mentioned above, two randomised trials proved the combination of trastuzumab with either paclitaxel (H0648g) [18] or docetaxel (M77001) [19] superior to chemotherapy alone. In H0648g, patients who had not received prior adjuvant anthracycline-based therapy were treated with a combination of doxorubicin and trastuzumab. While this combination again was highly effective in terms of oncological end points, a surprisingly high rate of cardiotoxicity was observed.

3 Trastuzumab in the Adjuvant Setting

Due to the proven benefits of trastuzumab in the palliative setting, adjuvant trials were initiated evaluating the possible role of trastuzumab in the prevention of breast cancer recurrences. More than 13,000 women were included in a total of six prospective randomised phase III trials. Five studies showed a benefit for the respective trastuzumab groups in terms of progression-free survival and (with the exception of the FinHER-trial) overall survival. Those results have ultimately established trastuzumab as golden standard in the adjuvant therapy for Her-2-positive early breast cancer. Importantly, chemotherapy regimens and the timing of trastuzumab administration varied among the different studies. Therefore, a number of unanswered questions concerning the optimal way to administer adjuvant trastuzumab remain. Furthermore, the last trial to report, the French PACS 04 study, presented divergent results: Herein, no additional benefit was found with the addition of adjuvant trastuzumab. Respective designs of the adjuvant breast cancer trials are summarised in Fig. 1.

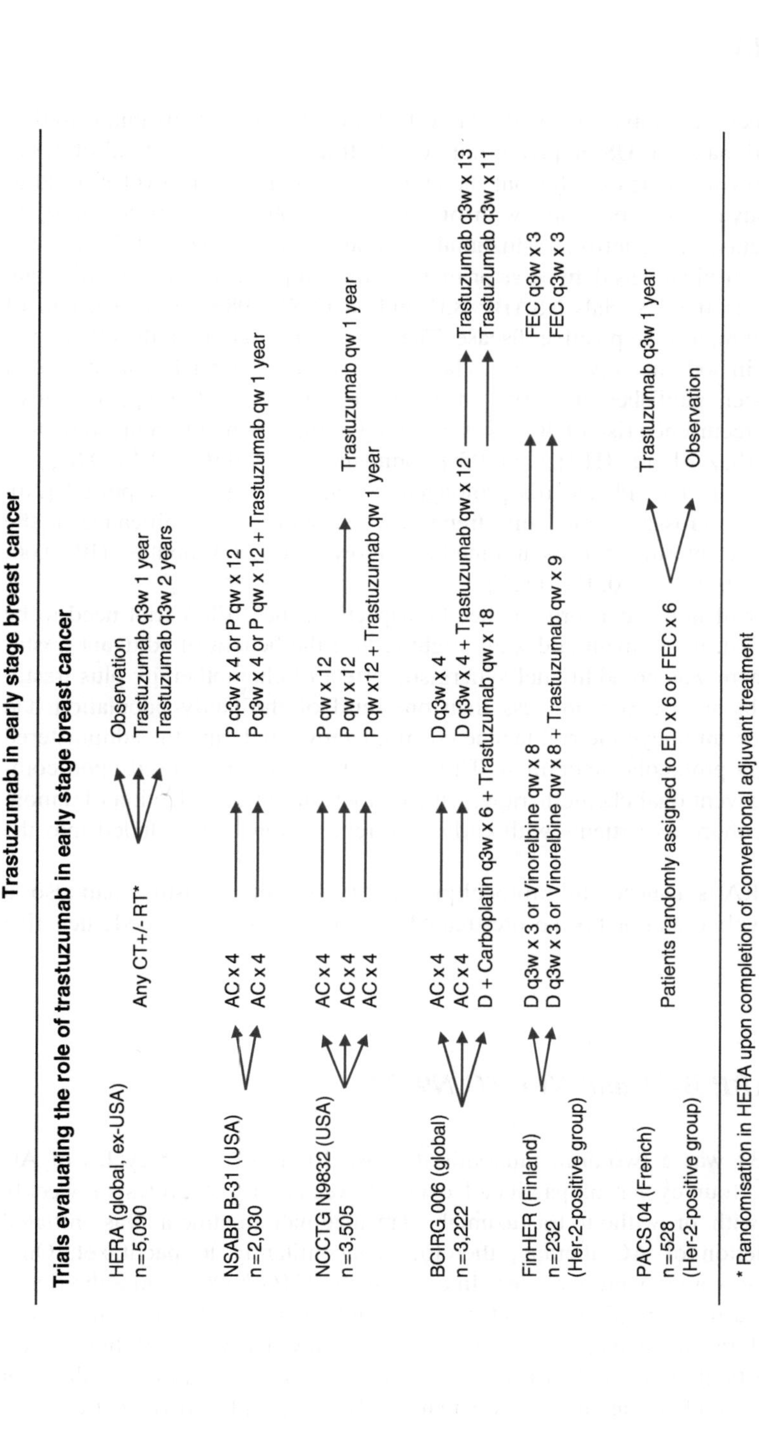

Fig. 1 *Trastuzumab in early stage breast cancer*. Abbreviations: *A* doxorubicin; *C* cyclophosphamide; *D* Docetaxel; *E* epidoxorubicin; *F* 5-FU; *P* paclitaxel; *q3w* every 3 weeks; *qw* weekly; *RT* radiotherapy

3.1 HERA

HERA (Herceptin Adjuvant) was the largest of the adjuvant trastuzumab studies. This international, non-US, adjuvant multicentre trial randomised a total of 5,102 patients following standard adjuvant therapy (a minimum of four cycles of adjuvant/neo-adjuvant chemotherapy with or without radiotherapy was required) to three treatment arms: Control, trastuzumab 12 months and trastuzumab 24 months. Disease-free survival was defined as primary study end point. It is noteworthy that in difference to the US-trials NSABP-B31 and NCCTG N9831, just over half of women had lymph-node positive disease. Therefore, information on the efficacy of trastuzumab in node-negative disease is largely derived from the HRA study. Initial data have been published in 2005. At 1 year of median follow-up, a relative reduction of recurrence risk of 46% was observed in the treatment group compared with control (hazard ratio [HR], 0.54; 95% confidence interval [CI], 0.43–0.67; $p <$ 0.0001). Further, a trend towards prolonged overall survival was reported [26]. Despite a 51% crossover rate, this trend reached statistical significance at the second planned interim analysis at a median follow-up of 23.5 months (HR, 0.66; 95% CI, 0.47–0.91; $p = 0.0115$) [27].

A number of issues concerning specific aspects of the HERA trial need to be discussed: First, the sequential design might reduce the benefit of adjuvant trastuzumab, as there was no additional synergistic effect of chemotherapy plus trastuzumab combinations. Second, less than one-third of the study population had received prior anthracycline and taxane chemotherapy, rendering the administered chemotherapy protocols suboptimal. Third, patients were randomised upon completion of conventional chemotherapy, which may result in the selection of a more favourable cohort, as patients with early recurrences were not included into the study.

Still, HERA is a successful protocol proving the benefit of trastuzumab also in non-anthracycline and/or taxane pre-treated patients as well as in node-negative tumours.

3.2 NSABP B-31 and NCCTG N9831

NSABP B-31 was a two-arm, randomised phase III trial of four cycles of AC followed by four cycles of paclitaxel every 3 weeks (or 12 cycles of weekly paclitaxel) with or without trastuzumab. Trastuzumab treatment was initiated after completion of AC therapy, therefore concomitantly to paclitaxel. Only node-positive women were included. In contrast, NCCTG N9831 had a three-arm design. Two arms were identical to the corresponding arms of B-31, while a third arm initiated trastuzumab after the end of chemotherapy (HERA style). In the latter trial, also patients with high-risk node-negative disease were allowed, although their relative number was much lower than in HERA. Similar to B-31, treatment again consisted of ACx4 followed by 12 cycles of weekly paclitaxel. Therefore, with FDA approval, a joint analysis comparing the two concurrent trastuzumab arms with the two control arms was conducted. A total number of 3,968 patients were included in the combined analysis, of which 93% had node-positive tumours.

After 2 years of median follow-up, patients treated with trastuzumab had a significantly longer disease-free survival as compared to the control group (HR, 0.48; 95% CI, 0.39–0.59; $p < 0.001$). Also, a significant benefit in terms of overall survival was observed (HR, 0.67; 95% CI, 0.48–0.93; $p = 0.015$) [28]. At a median follow-up of 2.9 years, despite a 21% crossover rate, updated results were similar: Risk of both, disease recurrence (HR, 0.48; 95% CI, 0.41–0.57; $p < 0.00001$) and death (HR, 0.65; 95% CI, 0.51–0.84; $p = 0.0007$) was significantly reduced [29].

Again, a number of aspects need to be considered. A small subsets of patients included in the joint analysis was identified Her-2-negative at central review. Furthermore, adjuvant AC→P might be considered a suboptimal adjuvant chemotherapy regimen.

3.3 BCIRG 006

A third trial was initiated by the BCIRG. This randomised three-arm open-label study conducted at centres in the US, Europe, South Africa, Asia and Venezuela had a slightly different design. Control arm consisted of ACx4 followed by four cycles of docetaxel every 3 weeks. This was compared to the same regimen plus trastuzumab (initiated after AC as in the North American studies) and a third (anthracycline-free) arm consisting of carboplatin, docetaxel and trastuzumab (TCH). A total of 3,222 patients were included, 71% had lymph-node-positive tumours.

Of interest is the inclusion of an anthracycline-free regimen. In the light of cardiac safety concerns, this seems an attractive option in patients with known pre-existing cardiac conditions. Currently however, anthracycline-free regimens cannot be considered a standard in the adjuvant therapy of breast cancer.

Updated results were presented at the 2006 San Antonio Breast Cancer Symposium [30]. At a median follow-up of 36 months, both trastuzumab groups were significantly superior over AC→docetaxel in terms of recurrence-free (HR, 0.61; 95% CI, 0.48–0.76; $p < 0.0001$ [AC→docetaxel+trastuzumab]; HR, 0.67; 95% CI, 0.54–0.83; $p = 0.0003$ [TCH]) as well as overall survival (HR, 0.59; 95% CI, 0.42–0.85; $p = 0.004$ [AC→docetaxel+trastuzumab]; HR, 0.66; 95% CI, 0.47–0.93; $p = 0.017$ [TCH]).

3.4 FinHER

A total of 1,010 women with node-positive or high-risk node-negative breast cancers were accrued to this randomised, controlled, open-label trial. The study was designed to compare the relative benefits of three cycles of docetaxel administered every 3 weeks to twelve cycles of weekly vinorelbine before receiving three cycles of FEC. Two hundred and thirty-two Her-2-positive patients were further randomised to nine cycles of weekly trastuzumab or control. Recurrence free survival was defined as primary end point.

While there was only a trend towards improved overall survival, a significant reduction in recurrence-free survival events was observed in patients receiving trastuzumab (HR, 0.42; 95% CI, 0.21–0.83; $p = 0.01$) [31]. In the overall population, docetaxel was significantly more active than vinorelbine in the adjuvant treatment of breast cancers.

This trial, while interesting, is limited by the small number of Her-2-positive patients as well as the non-significant improvement of overall survival. Therefore, further trials challenging the optimal duration of trastuzumab treatment must be awaited. For now, the golden standard remains treatment for 12 months.

3.5 PACS 04

This study is important, as it was the first – and hitherto only – trial not to report an additional benefit of trastuzumab. In total, 3,010 women with node-positive breast cancer were randomised to six cycles of epirubicin plus docetaxel or six cycles of FEC (epirubicin 100 mg/m^2). No results from this randomisation became available yet. The 528 Her-2-positive patients included were further randomised to trastuzumab for 1 year versus control upon availability of their respective Her-2-status. Similar to HERA, patients started trastuzumab after the completion of conventional adjuvant chemotherapy and irradiation.

At a median follow-up of 4 years, there was no added benefit observed for the addition of trastuzumab over chemotherapy alone in terms of recurrence-free survival (HR, 0.86; 95% CI, 0.61–1.22; $p = 0.41$) as well as overall survival (HR, 1.27; 95% CI, 0.68–2.38) [32].

While the study may be underpowered to detect a small advantage for the trastuzumab group, it may appear reasonable to ask whether the HERA-style sequential approach might have added to these results.

3.6 Discussion of Adjuvant Trials

When considering the above presented studies, despite PACS 04 results, there is clear-cut evidence in support of trastuzumab for 12 months in the adjuvant setting. Due to different designs of the adjuvant trials, a number of questions concerning the optimal use of trastuzumab remain unanswered.

In the light of BCIRG 006, it is intriguing to further evaluate the potential future role of an anthracycline-free regimen.

Also, the aspect of treatment duration is not resolved yet. While the HERA-trial evaluated longer treatment – the third arm (trastuzumab for 24 months) has not yet reported – FinHER is suggesting that less than 1 year of treatment might be sufficient. This question was also probed in E2198, a pilot trial examining the cardiac side effects of paclitaxel plus trastuzumab prior to doxorubicin plus cyclophosphamide (AC) in Her-2-positive patients. Patients received paclitaxel plus weekly trastuzumab for 10 weeks followed by four cycles of AC. Upon completion of chemotherapy, one arm received trastuzumab for a further 52 weeks. Disease-free survival and overall survival were comparable between the two groups. The authors concluded that while the trial was not designed or powered to test for non-inferiority of short-course trastuzumab, a significant advantage for prolonged trastuzumab administration was not observed. Currently, two major trials are ongoing directly comparing short- versus long-course therapy. Up until results from those studies become available, the matter is open to speculation and 12 months of adjuvant trastuzumab remains the golden standard.

Obviously, another important issue concerns the optimal time-point of trastuzumab initiation. In HERA and PACS 04, biological therapy was started upon completion of chemotherapy and irradiation. All other trials had a shorter or longer course of concurrent therapy. The obvious advantage of such a design is the minimisation of post-surgery trastuzumab delays (1–4 months versus 8 months in HERA) [11], furthermore, preclinical models had suggested a synergistic effect of trastuzumab when administered in conjunction with certain chemotherapeutic agents [13]. PACS 04, using a sequential design, indeed reported no benefit of trastuzumab. When considering the results of the above-mentioned studies, patients with early relapses, who are assumed to derive the largest benefit from concomitant treatment, were not included into the HERA study population due to the randomisation after the end of conventional therapy. This might have added to the positive results of the HERA trial. On the other hand, it is reasonable to assume that a longer time-span between anthracycline exposure and initiation of trastuzumab might reduce cardiac toxicity. It is hoped for that result from the sequential treatment arm of N9831 when available will provide further insight into the relative risks and benefits of the two different approaches.

Another largely unresolved question concerns the concurrent administration of trastuzumab with radiotherapy. Again, preclinical data suggest a radiosensitising effect of concurrent trastuzumab [33]. Currently, no data are available from prospective randomised studies. Yet, in a subgroup analysis of N9831 concurrent adjuvant radiotherapy and trastuzumab were not associated with increased acute adverse events, including cardiac side effects. Still, authors concluded that further follow-up is required to assess late adverse events [34]. Therefore, for the moment being, the combination of adjuvant irradiation and trastuzumab appears safe, and may enhance irradiation activity.

Only a very limited number of small-size tumours (pT1a, pT1b) were included in the above-mentioned trials. Therefore, it is not possible to give a final recommendation concerning those patients and chemotherapy plus trastuzumab may not be necessary in node-negative tumours smaller than 1 cm in size [35]. However, a combined retrospective analysis of approximately 1,000 women with tumours <1 cm suggests that even in this relative good-risk subgroup, Her-2-positive patients had 5.09 (95% CI, 2.56–10.14; $p < 0.0001$) times the risk of recurrence and 7.81 times (95% CI, 3.17–19.22; $p < 0.0001$) the risk of distant recurrence compared with patients with hormone receptor-positive tumours, leaving this matter to debate [36].

With the establishment of antibody therapy in early stage Her-2-positive breast cancer, recurrence rate was reduced by approximately 50%. Despite this success, a number of patients will still experience disease recurrence during antibody therapy or upon follow-up. Therefore, there is an urgent need to answer the question, whether trastuzumab should be re-induced in those individuals. Data from the RHEA (Re-treatment after Herceptin Adjuvant) phase II trial, which is currently ongoing, will hopefully provide information concerning this problem [37].

4 Trastuzumab in the Neo-adjuvant Setting

First reported in 1973 in inoperable breast cancer, the concept of pre-operative treatment has evolved into the use in operable disease with the objective of increasing the rate of breast conserving surgeries [38]. Different studies lead to the assumption that pathologic complete response (pCR) might act as surrogate for improved survival [39–41]. Due to the high efficacy of trastuzumab in the metastatic setting, it was reasonable to evaluate the effect on pCR in a neo-adjuvant setting. Early phase II trials reported pCR rates in the range of 18–39% [42–45].

In a phase III trial, patients received four cycles of paclitaxel every 3 weeks followed by four cycles of 5-FU, epirubicin and cyclophosphamide (FEC) with or without weekly trastuzumab for 24 weeks. The trial was terminated prematurely after the first 34 patients completed therapy, because a significant difference in terms of pCR favouring the trastuzumab arm was observed (66.7% versus 25%; $p = 0.02$) [46]. The German GeparQuattro trial randomised patients to four cycles of epirubicin plus cyclophosphamide (EC) followed by four cycles of docetaxel with or without capecitabine. Her-2-positive patients were treated with trastuzumab every 3 weeks concurrently to chemotherapy. pCR rates at surgery were 31.8% with trastuzumab and 15.4% without trastuzumab ($p < 0.001$). Importantly, none of the patients included on the trial experienced congestive heart failure or a decrease in left ventricular ejection fraction <45% [47]. The Austrian Breast and Colorectal Cancer Study Group (ABSCG) has now completed recruitment of ABSCG 24, a neo-adjuvant trial comparing six cycles of standard epirubicin plus docetaxel (ED) to ED with the addition of capecitabine. Her-2-positive patients had a further randomisation to trastuzumab versus control [37]. Results are not available yet, but are expected to be presented at the 2009 San Antonio Breast Cancer Symposium.

A meta-analysis of eight neo-adjuvant trials conducted by the German Breast Group and AGO (Arbeitsgemeinschaft Gynäkologische Onkologie; Working group Gynaecologic Oncology) included a total of 6,634 patients, 1,407 of which were Her-2-positive; 671 of those had received neo-adjuvant trastuzumab, while the remaining 736 had not. pCR rates reported were 41.1% in trastuzumab-treated patients, as compared to 27.7% [48].

While similar to the adjuvant setting the optimal combination of chemotherapy plus trastuzumab awaits further clarification, it appears reasonable to accept trastuzumab as golden standard even in the pre-operative setting.

5 Side Effects of Adjuvant Trastuzumab Therapy

The main issue of trastuzumab-related side effects regard cardiac toxicity. This problem was first reported in the pivotal metastatic trial, with the highest frequency in patients treated with a combination of doxorubicin plus trastuzumab [18]. In the adjuvant setting, approximately 5% of patients are expected to develop some form of cardiac function impairment, and 1% may develop symptomatic congestive heart failure (CHF) [26, 28, 49]. In most cases, the systolic dysfunction appears to be reversible [50], still, a close monitoring of patients on trastuzumab treatment is mandatory. At highest risk for a drop of left ventricular ejection fraction (LVEF) are patients of old age and those with known hypertension; further risk factors include pre-existing diabetes, coronary heart disease, and valvular dysfunction [11, 50].

When comparing the rates of cardiac dysfunction in HERA to results from the combined analysis of NSABP B-31 and NCCTG N9831, it is noteworthy that cardiac side effects appear less pronounced in the HERA study [51]. It is possible that the sequential design of HERA may hold responsible for this observation; furthermore, the number of patients receiving anthracyclines as adjuvant treatment was lower in the HERA study [11, 26]. Randomisation in HERA occurred upon completion of conventional treatment, and the eligibility threshold of LVEF was more stringent in HERA ($\geq$55% as compared to $\geq$50%) [51]. This might have excluded patients with worse LVEF, thereby apparently reducing cardiac side effects.

Further adverse events reported were mainly concerning anaphylactic reactions; furthermore, the HERA trial reported a minimal increase of infections (22 patients [1.3%] versus 7 patients [0.4%] in the control group) [26], and the combined analysis of NSABP B-31 and NCCTG N9831 trials observed rare cases of interstitial pneumonitis that in some cases appeared to be related to trastuzumab therapy (four cases in B-31 and five in N9831). In BCIRG 006, there were no significant differences in grade 3 or 4 haematologic or non-haematological adverse events among the three treatment arms [52]. Also, in the FinHER trial, no differences were observed in the respective trastuzumab and non-trastuzumab groups [31]. Interestingly, a recently published paper evaluated gastrointestinal side effects of trastuzumab (i.e. nausea, vomiting, diarrhoea, abdominal pain). Those were observed in as much as 12% of trastuzumab administrations. As only 46 patients were available for this retrospective chart review, however, further prospective evaluation of those symptoms appears necessary [53]. A single case report is available describing a case of trastuzumab-induced hepatopathy in an otherwise healthy women receiving adjuvant therapy for breast cancer [54]. This report, however, has not been verified in prospective studies.

6 Ongoing Studies

Lapatinib is an orally available tyrosine kinase inhibitor blocking the tyrosine kinase domains of EGFR and Her-2. Lapatinib in combination with capecitabine was found superior over chemotherapy alone in terms of response rate and progression-free survival [55]. Furthermore, patients in the combination group experienced significantly less brain metastases. This is mirrored by another trial suggesting direct activity of lapatinib on cerebral lesions [56].

In the adjuvant setting, the ALLTO trial (BIG 2-06/N063D; NCT00490139) is currently ongoing. This prospective randomised phase III study incorporates four treatment arms: A standard arm of trastuzumab for 1 year is compared with lapatinib for 1 year, lapatinib for 12 weeks followed by trastuzumab for 6 months (sequential) or trastuzumab in combination with lapatinib (concurrent). Recruitment is well on the way, and study completion is expected for June 2010 [37].

Bevacizumab is a humanised monoclonal antibody targeting vascular endothelial growth factor (VEGF). Increased signalling via the ras/raf/MAPKinase signalling pathway, as is the case in Her-2-positive disease, will increase HIF-1α and consequently VEGF [57–60]. This mechanism may be blocked by trastuzumab. Based upon this rationale, a randomised multicentre study is currently on the way, evaluating docetaxel plus trastuzumab with or without bevacizumab in the first line metastatic setting (AVAREL; A Study of Avastin (Bevacizumab) in Combination With Herceptin (Trastuzumab/Docetaxel) in Patients With HER-2-Positive Metastatic Breast Cancer; NCT00391092) [37]. Meanwhile, a randomised adjuvant study was initiated (BETH; Bevacizumab and Trastuzumab Adjuvant Therapy in Her-2-positive Breast Cancer; NCT00625898) [37].

Other important studies were mentioned already: The SOLD (Synergism or Long Duration; NCT00593697) and PHARE (Protocol of Herceptin Adjuvant with Reduced Exposure; NCT00381901) studies are directly comparing long-versus short-term trastuzumab treatment [37]. In this context, results from the 2-year trastuzumab arm of the HERA trial are also eagerly awaited. NCCTG N9831 again will hopefully resolve questions regarding the superiority of a concomitant versus a sequential approach for administering chemotherapy and trastuzumab. The RHEA trial is challenging the problem of trastuzumab re-induction in patients who progressed after adjuvant trastuzumab therapy.

7 Conclusion

Targeting Her-2 with trastuzumab has dramatically changed the prognosis of patients with Her-2-positive breast cancer, both in advanced and in early stage disease. Meanwhile, three prospective randomised phase III trials have reported superior overall survival when trastuzumab is added to conventional chemotherapy.

Still, questions remain concerning the potential role of anthracycline-free chemotherapy regimens (which might reduce cardiac toxicity), the optimal time point of trastuzumab initiation, the combination of trastuzumab and irradiation, the role of trastuzumab in tumours smaller than 1 cm and the optimal duration of trastuzumab therapy. A number of important trials are still ongoing and will hopefully resolve some of those questions.

References

1. American Cancer Society (2009) American Cancer Society Statistics 2009. Available at http://www.cancer.org/downloads/STT/Global_Facts_and_Figures_2007_rev2.pdf. Accessed 13 Aug 2009
2. Beatson GT (1896) On the treatment of inoperable causes of carcinoma of the mamma: suggestions for a new method of treatment with illustrative cases. Lancet 2:104–107
3. Slamon DJ, Clark GM, Wong SG, Levin WJ, Ullrich A, McGuire WL (1987) Human breast cancer: correlation of relapse and survival with amplification of the HER2/neu oncogene. Science 235:177–182
4. Paik S, Hazan R, Fisher ER, Sass RE, Fisher B, Redmond C, Schlessinger J, Lippman ME, King CR (1990) Pathologic finding from the National Surgical Adjuvant Breast and Bowel Project: prognostic significance of erbB-2 protein expression in primary breast cancer. J Clin Oncol 8:103–112
5. Kallioniemi OP, Holli K, Visakorpi T, Koivula T, Helin HH, Isola JJ (1991) Association of c-erbB-2 protein over-expression with high rate of cell proliferation, increased risk of visceral metastasis and poor long-term survival in breast cancer. Int J Cancer 4:650–655
6. Casalini P, Iorio MV, Galmozzi E, Ménard S (2004) Role of HER receptors family in development and differentiation. J Cell Physiol 200:343–350
7. Fukazawa R, Miller TA, Kuramochi Y, Frantz S, Kim YD, Marchionni MA, Kelly RA, Sawyer DB (2003) Neuregulin-1 protects ventricular myocytes from anthracycline-induced apoptosis via erbB4-dependent activation of PI3-kinase/Akt. J Mol Cell Cardiol 35:1473–1479
8. Denoux Y, Arnould L, Fiche M, Lannes B, Couturier J, Vincent-Salomon A, Penault-Llorca F, Antoine M, Balaton A, Baranzelli MC, Becette V et al (2003) HER2 gene amplification assay: is CISH an alternative to FISH? Ann Pathol 22:617–622
9. Gjierdrum L, Sorensen B, Kjeldsen E, Sorensen FB, Nexo E, Hamilton-Dutoit S (2004) Real-time quantitative PCR of microdissected paraffin-embedded breast carcinoma: an alternative method for HER-2/neu analysis. J Mol Diagn 6:42–51
10. Paik S, Kim C, Wolmark N (2008) Her2 status and benefit from adjuvant trastuzumab in breast cancer. N Engl J Med 358:1409–1411
11. Mackey J, McLeod D, Ragaz J, Gelmon K, Verma S, Pritchard K, Laing K, Provencher L, Charbonneau LF (2009) Adjuvant targeted therapy in early breast cancer. Cancer 115:1154–1168

12. Nahta R, Yu D, Hung MC, Hortobagyi GN, Esteva FJ (2006) Mechanisms of disease: understanding resistance to Her2-targeted therapy in human breast cancer. Nat Clin Pract Oncol 3:269–280
13. Pegram M, Hsu S, Lewis G, Pietras R, Beryt M, Sliwkowski M, Coombs D, Baly D, Kabbinavar F, Slamon D (1999) Inhibitory effects of combinations of HER2/neu antibody and chemotherapeutic agents used for treatment of human breast cancers. Oncogene 18:2241–2251
14. Scaltriti M, Verma C, Guzman M, Jimenez J, Parra JL, Pedersen K, Smith DJ, Landolfi S, Ramon y Cajal S, Arribas J, Baselga J (2009) Lapatinib, a HER2 tyrosine kinase inhibitor, induces stabilization and accumulation of HER2 and potentiates trastuzumab-dependent cell cytotoxicity. Oncogene 28:803–814
15. O'Shaugnessy J, Blackwell KL, Burstein H, Storniolo AM, Sledge G, Baselga J, Koehler M, Laabs S, Florance A, Roychowdhury D (2008) A randomized study of lapatinib alone or in combination with trastuzumab in heavily pretreated HER2+ metastatic breast cancer progressing on trastuzumab therapy. J Clin Oncol 26(Suppl 17):154S
16. Baselga J, Tripathy D, Mendelsohn J, Baughman S, Benz CC, Dantis L, Sklarin NT, Seidman AD, Hudis CA, Moore J, Rosen PP, Twaddell T, Henderson IC, Norton L (1996) Phase II study of weekly intravenous recombinant humanized anti-p185HER2 monoclonal antibody in patients with HER2/neu-overexpressing metastatic breast cancer. J Clin Oncol 14:737–744
17. Cobleigh MA, Vogel CL, Tripathy D, Robert NJ, Scholl S, Fehrenbacher L, Wolter JM, Paton V, Shak S, Lieberman G, Slamon DJ (1999) Multinational study of the efficacy and safety of humanized anti-HER2 monoclonal antibody in women who have HER2-overexpressing metastatic breast cancer that has progressed after chemotherapy for metastatic disease. J Clin Oncol 17:2639–2648
18. Slamon DJ, Leyland-Jones B, Shak S, Fuchs H, Paton V, Bajamonde A, Fleming T, Eiermann W, Wolter J, Pegram M, Baselga J, Norton L (2001) Use of chemotherapy plus a monoclonal antibody against HER2 for metastatic breast cancer that overexpresses HER2. N Engl J Med 344:783–792
19. Marty M, Cognetti F, Maraninchi D, Snyder R, Mauriac L, Tubiana-Hulin M, Chan S, Grimes D, Antón A, Lluch A et al (2005) Randomized phase II trial of the efficacy and safety of trastuzumab combined with docetaxel in patients with human epidermal growth factor 2-positive metastatic breast cancer administered as first-line treatment: the M77001 study group. J Clin Oncol 23:4265–4274
20. Vogel CL, Cobleigh MA, Tripathy D, Gutheil JC, Harris LN, Fehrenbacher L, Slamon DJ, Murphy M, Novotny WF, Burchmore M et al (2002) Efficacy and safety of trastuzumab as a single agent in first-line treatment of HER2-overexpressing metastatic breast cancer. J Clin Oncol 20:719–726
21. Lu Y, Zi X, Zhao Y, Mascarenhas D, Pollak M (2001) Insulin-like growth factor-I receptor signaling and resistance to trastuzumab (Herceptin). J Natl Cancer Inst 93:1852–1857
22. Nagata Y, Lan KH, Zhou X, Tan M, Esteva FJ, Sahin AA, Klos KS, Li P, Monia BP, Nguyen NT, Hortobagyi GN, Hung MC, Yu D (2004) PTEN activation contributes to tumor inhibition by trastuzumab, and loss of PTEN predicts trastuzumab resistance in patients. Cancer Cell 6:117–127
23. Clark AS, West K, Streicher S, Dennis PA (2002) Constitutive and inducible Akt activity promotes resistance to chemotherapy, trastuzumab, or tamoxifen in breast cancer cells. Mol Cancer Ther 1:707–717
24. Migliaccio I, Gutierrez MC, Wu MF, Wu M-F, Wong H, Pavlick A, Hilsenbeck SG, Horlings HM, Rimawi M, Berns K et al (2009) PI3 kinase activation and response to trastuzumab or lapatinib in HER-2 overexpressing locally advanced breast cancer (LABC). Cancer Res 69 (suppl 2):72S
25. Esparís-Ogando A, Díaz-Rodríguez E, Pandiella A (1999) Signaling-competent truncated forms of ErbB2 in breast cancer cells: differential regulation by protein kinase C and phosphatidylinositol 3-kinase. Biochem J 344:339–348

26. Piccart-Gebhart MJ, Procter M, Leyland-Jones B, Goldhirsch A, Untch M, Smith I, Gianni L, Baselga J, Bell R, Jackisch C et al (2005) Trastuzumab after adjuvant chemotherapy in HER2-positive breast cancer. N Engl J Med 353:1659–1672
27. Smith I, Procter M, Gelber RD, Guillaume S, Feyereislova A, Dowsett M, Goldhirsch A, Untch M, Mariani G, Baselga J et al (2007) Two year follow-up of trastuzumab after adjuvant chemotherapy in Her2-positive breast cancer: a randomised controlled trial. Lancet 369:29–36
28. Romond EH, Perez EA, Bryant J, Suman VJ, Geyer CE Jr, Davidson NE, Tan-Chiu E, Martino S, Paik S, Kaufman PA et al (2005) Trastuzumab plus adjuvant chemotherapy for operable HER2-positive breast cancer. N Engl J Med 353:1673–1684
29. Perez EA, Romond EH, Suman VJ, Jeong J, Davidson NE, Geyer CE, Martino S, Mamounas EP, Kauffman PA, Wolmark N, NCCTG/NSABP (2007) Updated results of the combined analysis of NCCTG N9831and NSABP B-31 adjuvant chemotherapy with/without trastuzumab in patients with her2-positve breast cancer. J Clin Oncol 25(Suppl 18):6S
30. Slamon D, Eiermann W, Robert N, Pienkowski T, Martin M, Pawlicki M, Chan A, Smylie M, Liu M, Falkson C et al (2006) BCIRG 006: 2nd interim analysis phase III randomized trial comparing doxorubicin and cyclophosphamide followed by docetaxel (AC→T) with doxorubicin and cyclophosphamide followed by docetaxel and trastuzumab (AC→TH) with docetaxel, carboplatin and trastuzumab (TCH) in Her2neu positive early breast cancer patients. Breast Cancer Res Treat 100(Suppl 1):abstract 52
31. Joensuu H, Kellokumpu-Lehtinen P-L, Bono P, Alanko T, Kataja V, Asola R, Utriainen T, Kokko R, Hemminki A, Tarkkanen M et al (2006) Adjuvant docetaxel or vinorelbine with or without trastuzumab for breast cancer. N Engl J Med 354:809–820
32. Spielmann M, Roché H, Humblet Y, Delozier T, Bourgeois H, Serin D, Romieu G, Canon JL, Monnier A, Piot G et al (2007) 3-Year follow-up of trastuzumab following adjuvant chemotherapy in node positive HER2-positive breast cancer patients: results of the PACS-04 trial. Breast Cancer Res Treat 106(suppl 1):19S
33. Liang K, Lu Y, Jin W, Ang KK, Milas L, Fan Z (2003) Sensitization of breast cancer cells to radiation by trastuzumab. Mol Cancer Ther 2:1113–1120
34. Halyard MY, Pisansky TM, Dueck AC, Suman V, Pierce L, Solin L, Marks L, Davidson N, Martino S, Kaufman P et al (2009) Radiotherapy and adjuvant trastuzumab in operable breast cancer: tolerability and adverse event data from the NCCTG Phase III Trial N9831. J Clin Oncol 27:2638–2644
35. Goldhirsch A, Wood WC, Gelber RD, Coates AS, Thürlimann B, Senn HJ (2007) 10th St. Gallen conference; Progress and promise: highlights of the international expert consensus on the primary therapy of early breast cancer 2007. Ann Oncol 18:1133–1144
36. Rakkhit R, Broglio K, Peintinger F, Cardoso F, Hanrahan EO, Litton JK, Sahin A, Larsimont D, Meric-Bernstam F, Buchholz TA et al (2008) Significant increased recurrence rates among breast cancer patients with HER2-positive tumors 1 cm or smaller. Cancer Res 69 (Suppl 2):97S
37. ClinicalTrials. Available at http://www.clinicaltrials.gov. Accessed 13 Aug 2009
38. Buzdar AU (2007) Preoperative chemotherapy treatment of breast cancer – a review. Cancer 110:2394–2407
39. Bear HD, Anderson S, Smith RE, Geyer CE Jr, Mamounas EP, Fisher B, Brown AM, Robidoux A, Margolese R, Kahlenberg MS et al (1999) Sequential preoperative or postoperative docetaxel added to preoperative doxorubicin plus cyclophosphamide for operable breast cancer: National Surgical Breast and Bowel Project B-27. J Clin Oncol 24:2019–2027
40. Kuerer HM, Newman LA, Smith TL, Ames FC, Hunt KK, Dhingra K, Theriault RL, Singh G, Binkley SM, Sneige N et al (1999) Clinical course of breast cancer patients with complete pathologic primary tumor and axillary lymph node response to doxorubicin-based neoadjuvant chemotherapy. J Clin Oncol 17:460–469
41. Wolmark N, Wang J, Mamounas E, Bryant J, Fisher B (2001) Preoperative chemotherapy in patients with operable breast cancer: 9-year results from National Surgical Breast and Bowel Project B-18. J Natl Cancer Inst 30:96–102

42. Wenzel C, Hussian D, Bartsch R, Pluschnig U, Locker GJ, Rudas M, Gnant MF, Jakesz R, Zielinkski CC, Steger GG (2004) Preoperative therapy with epidoxorubicin and docetaxel plus trastuzumab in patients with primary breast cancer: a pilot study. J Cancer Res Clin Oncol 130:400–404
43. Burstein H, Harris L, Gelman R, Lester SC, Nunes RA, Kaelin CM, Parker LM, Ellisen LW, Kuter I, Gadd MA et al (2003) Preoperative therapy with trastuzumab and paclitaxel followed by sequential adjuvant doxorubicin/cyclophosphamide for HER2 overexpressing stage II or III breast cancer: a pilot study. J Clin Oncol 21:46–53
44. Jahanzeb M, Brufsky A, Erban J, Lewis D, Limentani S (2005) Dose-dense neoadjuvant treatment of women with breast cancer utilizing docetaxel, vinorelbine and trastuzumab with growth factor support. J Clin Oncol 23(Suppl 16):16S
45. Hurley J, Doliny P, Reis I, Silva O, Gomez-Fernandez C, Velez P, Pauletti G, Powell JE, Pegram MD, Slamon DJ (2006) Docetaxel, cisplatin, and trastuzumab as primary systemic therapy for human epidermal growth factor receptor 2-positive locally advanced breast cancer. J Clin Oncol 24:1831–1838
46. Buzdar A, Ibrahim N, Francis D, Booser DJ, Thomas ES, Theriault RL, Pusztai L, Green MC, Arun BK, Giordano SH et al (2005) Significantly higher pathologic complete remission rate after neoadjuvant therapy with trastuzumab, paclitaxel, and epirubicin chemotherapy: results of a randomized trial in human epidermal growth factor receptor 2-positive operable breast cancer. J Clin Oncol 23:3676–3685
47. Von Minckwitz G, Rezai M, Loibl S, Fasching PA, Juober J, Tesch H, Bauerfeind I, Hilfrich J, Mehta K, Untch M (2008) Effect of trastuzumab on pathologic complete response rate of neoadjuvant EC-docetaxel treatment in Her2-overexpressing breast cancer: results of the phase III GeparQuattro study. Abstract 226. Presented at the 2008 ASCO Breast Cancer Symposium
48. Von Minckwitz G, Kaufmann M, Kümmel S, Fasching P, Eiermann W, Blohmer J-U, Costa SD, Sibylle L, Dietmar V, Untch M (2009) Integrated meta-analysis on 6402 patients with early breast cancer receiving neoadjuvant anthracycline-taxane +/− trastuzumab containing chemotherapy. Cancer Res 69(suppl 2):82S
49. Perez EA, Rodeheffer R (2004) Clinical cardiac tolerability of trastuzumab. J Clin Oncol 22:322–329
50. Guarneri V, Lenihan DJ, Valero V, Durand JB, Broglio K, Hess KR, Michaud LB, Gonzalez-Angulo AM, Hortobagyi GN, Esteva FJ (2006) Long-term cardiac tolerability of trastuzumab in metastatic breast cancer: The M.D. Anderson Cancer Center experience. J Clin Oncol 24:4107–4115
51. Madarnas Y, Trudeau M, Franek JA, McCready D, Pritchard KI, Messersmith H (2008) Adjuvant/neoadjuvant trastuzumab therapy in women with HER-2/neu-overexpressing breast cancer: a systematic review. Cancer Treat Rev 34:539–557
52. Slamon D, Eierman W, Robert N, Pienkowski T, Martin M, Pawlicki M, Chan M, Smylie M, Liu M, Falkson C et al (2005) Phase III randomized trial comparing doxorubicin and cyclophosphamide followed by docetaxel (AC→T) with doxorubicin and cyclophosphamide followed by docetaxel and trastuzumab (AC→TH) with docetaxel, carboplatin and trastuzumab (TCH) in HER2 positive early breast cancer patients: BCIRG 006 study. Breast Can Res Treat 94(suppl 1):5S
53. Al-Dasooqi N, Bowen JM, Gibson RJ, Sullivan T, Lees J, Keefe DM (2009) Trastuzumab induces gastrointestinal side effects in Her2-overexpressing breast cancer patients. Invest New Drugs 27:173–178
54. Srinivasan S, Parsa V, Liu CY, Fontana JA (2008) Trastuzumab-induced hepatotoxicity. Ann Pharmacother 42:1497–1501
55. Geyer CE, Forster J, Lindquist D, Chan S, Romieu CG, Pienkowski T, Jagiello-Gruszfeld A, Crown J, Chan A, Kaufman B (2006) Lapatinib plus capecitabine for HER2-positive advanced breast cancer. N Engl J Med 355:2733–2743
56. Lin NU, Carey LA, Liu MC, Younger J, Come SE, Ewend M, Harris GJ, Bullitt E, Van den Abbeele AD et al (2006) Phase II trial of lapatinib for brain metastases in patients with

human epidermal growth factor receptor 2-positive breast cancer. J Clin Oncol 26: 1993–1999
57. Laughner E, Taghavi P, Chiles K, Mahon PC, Semenza GL (2001) HER2 (neu) signaling increases the rate hypoxia-inducible factor 1α (HIF-1α) synthesis: novel mechanism for HIF-1-mediated vascular endothelial growth factor expression. Mol Cell Biol 21:3995–4004
58. Yen L, You XL, Al Moustafa AE, Batist G, Hynes NE, Mader S, Meloche S, Alaoui-Jamali MA (2000) Heregulin selectively upregulates vascular endothelial growth factor secretion in cancer cell and stimulates angiogenesis. Oncogene 19:3460–3469
59. Izumi Y, Xu L, di Tomaso E, Fukumura D, Jain RK (2002) Tumor biology: Herceptin acts as an anti-angiogenic cocktail. Nature 416:279–280
60. Konecny GE, Meng YG, Untch M, Wang HJ, Bauerfeind I, Epstein M, Stieber P, Vernes JM, Gutierrez J, Hong K et al (2004) Association between HER-2/neu and vascular endothelial growth factor expression predicts clinical outcome in primary breast cancer patients. Clin Cancer Res 10:1706–1716

Trastuzumab Resistance in Breast Cancer

Floriana Morgillo, Michele Orditura, Teresa Troiani, Erika Martinelli, Ferdinando De Vita, and Fortunato Ciardiello

Abstract The amplification and expression of ERBB2 have been linked with prognosis and response to therapy with the anti-HER-2-humanised monoclonal antibody, trastuzumab, in patients with advanced metastatic breast cancer. However, one of the major clinical problems encountered with trastuzumab treatment is that metastatic breast cancer patients, who initially responded to trastuzumab, showed disease progression within 1 year from treatment initiation. Several studies have already reported or speculated on potential mechanisms of resistance to trastuzumab. Despite these important leads, there is/are no biomarker(s) that can reliably predict lack of benefit from trastuzumab, which in turn can be used for subsequent clinical trial development and/or individual therapeutic decisions.

1 Introduction

The ErbB/HER family is composed of four growth factor receptors that share a high degree of sequence homology: EGFR (or erbB1 or HER1), erbB2 (or HER-2; or neu in rodents), erbB3 (or HER3) and erbB4 (or HER4). It has been well established that signalling through EGFR, HER-2, and HER3 is associated with malignant transformation and cancer progression by increasing proliferation, survival, metastasis and resistance to antitumour therapy [1]. These receptors are transmembrane proteins with intracellular tyrosine kinase activity (except for HER3), and their activation results from the formation of homodimers and heterodimers, which is dependent on their ligands (except for HER-2). The extracellular domain of HER-2 is unable to bind extracellular ligand and depends on heterodimerising with other ligand-activated receptors. Moreover, its catalytic activity can potently amplify signalling by ErbB-containing heterodimers via

F. Ciardiello (✉)
Oncologia Medica, Dipartimento di Internistica clinica e sperimentale "F. Magrassi A. Lanzara"
Seconda Università degli studi di Napoli, Via Sergio Pansini 5, 80131 Napoli, Italy
e-mail: fortunato.ciardiello@unina2.it

M. Sibilia et al. (eds.), *Drugs for HER-2-positive Breast Cancer*,
Milestones in Drug Therapy, DOI 10.1007/978-3-0346-0094-1_3,

increasing ligand binding affinity and/or receptor recycling and stability [1]. The localisation of HER-2 in epithelial cells is regulated by the membrane-associated glycoprotein MUC4 and sialomucin complex, indicating a critical role of MUC4 as an intramembrane modulator of HER-2 activity [2]. HER3 is deficient in tyrosine kinase activity and needs to bind other receptors of this family for enzyme function [1]. Interestingly, the association of kinase-dead HER3 with ligand-less HER-2, however, makes a remarkably efficient signalling complex, mediating multiple cellular function [3]. Over-expression of HER-2 leads to activation of the HER-2-mediated signalling pathway, even in the absence of ligand. HER-2 co-operating with other receptors mediates multiple downstream signalling pathways, including the mitogen-activated protein kinase (MAPK) and phosphatidylinositol-3-kinase (PI3K) pathways. These pathways are regulated by many HER-2 molecular partners, including Shc, Grb2, the Crk family of adaptor proteins, phospholipase Cγ, and the repressors of signalling, CHK and Dok-2 [1]. These signalling pathways play a key role in tumourigenesis by promoting cell proliferation, differentiation, angiogenesis, invasion and survival [1]. Moreover, nuclear expression of HER-2 has been significantly correlated with Cox-2 expression [4]. The contribution of nuclear HER-2 to the tumourigenic process clearly deserves further investigation.

EGFR is over-expressed in 20–30% of breast cancers occurring more frequently in triple-negative breast cancers (pathologically negative for oestrogen receptor, progesterone receptor and HER-2). Its over-expression predicts resistance to anti-oestrogen therapy in oestrogen receptor-positive breast indicating an aggressive cancer type and, consequently, poor prognosis [5]. A novel molecular classification established by DNA microarray technology and gene-expression profiles has identified HER-2 as an independent breast cancer subgroup [6], which has diagnostic, prognostic and therapeutic implications. HER-2 is over-expressed in 15–25% of invasive breast carcinomas, and this over-expression is due to gene amplification in more than 90% of cases [7].

Other mechanisms of hyperactivation include decreased levels of phosphatase, increased co-expression of other ErbB/HER receptors and/or their ligands (e.g. TGF-α and amphiregulin), heterodimerisation and crosstalk with other tyrosine kinases (e.g. IGF-IR) and interactions with the ER .

HER3 and HER4 are not considered strong prognostic markers in breast cancer. According to the above concept, all ErbB/HER family members work together, and alterations in one member have direct effects on the tightly controlled signalling pathway.

2 Trastuzumab: Clinical Efficacy and Resistance

Trastuzumab (Herceptin®; Genentech, South San Francisco, CA, USA) is a humanised monoclonal IgG1 that binds to the ectodomain of HER-2 and induces clinical responses in HER-2-over-expressing breast cancers prolonging patient survival when combined with chemotherapy [8, 9]. Trastuzumab has been the first HER-2-targeted therapy approved by the United States Food and Drug Administration (FDA) for the treatment of HER-2-over-expressing metastatic breast cancer (MBC). The clinical efficacy of trastuzumab seems limited to breast cancers that over-express HER-2 as measured by intense membrane staining in the majority of tumour cells with HER-2 antibodies (3+ by immunohistochemistry) or excess copies of the HER-2 gene determined by fluorescence in situ hybridisation. In addition, trastuzumab with adjuvant chemotherapy (either in sequence or in combination) significantly improves disease-free and overall survival rates in patients with early stage HER-2-over-expressing breast cancer [8–10]. Trastuzumab reduces signalling mediated by HER-2 through the phosphatidylinositol 3-kinase (PI3K) and mitogen-activated protein kinase (MAPK) cascades. Reduced downstream signalling through these pathways induces the cyclin-dependent kinase inhibitor p27kip1, which promotes cell cycle arrest and apoptosis [11]. Trastuzumab rapidly dissociates the non-receptor tyrosine kinase Src from HER-2, reducing Src activity such that the phosphatase and tensin homologue deleted on chromosome ten (PTEN) is dephosphorylated and translocated to the plasma membrane where it is active [12]. The efficacy of trastuzumab may also depend upon its ability to induce an immune response. HER-2-targeted antibodies, including trastuzumab, were shown to promote apoptosis in multiple breast cancer cell lines via antibody-dependent cellular cytotoxicity (ADCC) [13]. Trastuzumab has also been shown to inhibit angiogenesis, resulting in decreased microvessel density in vivo and reduced endothelial cell migration in vitro. Expression of pro-angiogenic factors was reduced, while expression of anti-angiogenic factors was increased in trastuzumab-treated tumours relative to control-treated tumours in vivo [14]. Combining trastuzumab with the chemotherapeutic agent paclitaxel actually inhibited angiogenesis more potently than did trastuzumab alone [15], perhaps due to trastuzumab-mediated normalisation of the tumour vasculature allowing for better drug delivery. However, many patients with HER-2 gene-amplified metastatic breast cancers do not respond or eventually escape trastuzumab, suggesting both de novo and acquired mechanisms of therapeutic resistance.

In fact, the rate of primary resistance to single-agent trastuzumab for HER-2-over-expressing MBC is 66–88% [16]. Further phase III trials revealed that combining trastuzumab with paclitaxel or docetaxel [17–19] could increase response rates, time to disease progression and overall survival compared with trastuzumab monotherapy. However, the majority of patients who achieve an initial response to trastuzumab-based regimens develop resistance within 1 year. In the adjuvant setting, administration of trastuzumab in combination with or following chemotherapy improves the disease-free and overall survival rates in patients with early stage breast cancer. However, approximately 15% of these women still develop metastatic disease despite trastuzumab-based adjuvant chemotherapy.

Elucidating the molecular mechanisms underlying primary or acquired (treatment-induced) trastuzumab resistance is critical to improving the survival of metastatic breast cancer patients whose tumours over-express HER-2 [20].

3 Trastuzumab: Mechanisms of Resistance

3.1 Steric Hindrance of Receptor–Antibody Interaction: Over-expression of MUC4

The first investigated mechanism by which resistance to targeted antibodies may develop was the disruption of the interaction between the therapeutic agent and the target protein. Resistance to trastuzumab was associated with increased expression of the membrane-associated glycoprotein MUC4 [21]. MUC4 was shown to bind and sterically hinder HER-2 from binding to trastuzumab [21, 22]. MUC4 has been suggested to contribute to cancer because of its ability to inhibit immune recognition of cancer cells, promote tumour progression and metastasis, suppress apoptosis and activate HER-2 [23]. MUC4 interacts directly with HER-2, an event that is dependent upon an epidermal growth factor (EGF)-like domain on the ASGP-2 subunit of MUC4 [21]. Through this interaction, it is proposed that MUC4 serves as a ligand for HER-2, resulting in increased phosphorylation of HER-2 on the residue Tyr1248, which is a major phosphorylation site contributing to the transforming ability of the HER-2 oncoprotein. MUC4 does not affect total HER-2 receptor expression levels [21]. In the JIMT-1 trastuzumab-resistant cell line described by Nagy and colleagues [22] established from a breast cancer patient showing *her-2* gene amplification and primary resistance to trastuzumab, the level of MUC4 protein was inversely correlated with the trastuzumab binding capacity, and knock-down of MUC4 increased the sensitivity of JIMT-1 cells to trastuzumab [22]. The conclusion was that elevated MUC4 expression masks the trastuzumab binding epitopes of HER-2, resulting in steric hindrance of the interaction between this antibody and its therapeutic target, resulting in drug resistance. Of interest, HER-2 at the same time is unable to interact with other proteins, such as EGFR or HER3, because of epitope masking by MUC4.

3.2 PTEN and PI3K Signalling

Growth factor receptor tyrosine kinases, such as HER-2 and IGF-IR, activate the PI3K signalling pathway. Constitutive PI3K/Akt activity was previously shown to inhibit cell-cycle arrest and apoptosis mediated by trastuzumab [24]. Indeed, trastuzumab-resistant cells derived from the BT474 HER-2-over-expressing breast cancer line demonstrated elevated levels of phosphorylated Akt and Akt kinase activity compared with parental cells [25]. These resistant cells also showed increased sensitivity to LY294002, a small molecule inhibitor of PI3K. Nagata and colleagues [12] provided compelling evidence supporting a role for the PI3K/Akt pathway in trastuzumab resistance. They demonstrated that decreased levels of the PTEN phosphatase resulted in increased PI3K/Akt phosphorylation and signalling and blocked trastuzumab-mediated growth arrest of HER-2-over-expressing breast cancer cells. Moreover, patients with PTEN-deficient HER-2-over-expressing breast tumours have a much poorer response to trastuzumab-based therapy and in PTEN-deficient cells, PI3K inhibitors rescued trastuzumab resistance in vitro and in vivo. These results suggest that PTEN loss may serve as a predictor of trastuzumab resistance, and that PI3K inhibitors or inhibitors of other downstream targets of PI3K signal, such as mTOR, should be explored as potential therapies in patients with trastuzumab-resistant tumours expressing low levels of PTEN protein.

3.3 Serum HER-2 Extracellular Domain

The full-length 185 kDa HER-2 protein has been reported to be cleaved by matrix metalloproteases into a 110 kDa extracellular domain (ECD), which is released into cell culture media [26] or circulating in serum in vivo [27], and a 95 kDa amino-terminally truncated membrane-associated fragment with increased kinase activity. The problem is that HER-2-targeted monoclonal antibodies bound to circulating ECD, competing away binding to membrane-bound HER-2. Hence, signalling from the receptor form of HER-2 continued in the presence of HER-2 antibodies, indicating that HER-2 ECD promoted resistance to HER-2-targeted antibody therapy.

Indeed, elevated serum levels of HER-2 ECD correlate with poor prognosis in patients with advanced breast cancer [27]. HER-2 over-expression in breast cancers correlated with elevated pre-treatment levels of circulating HER-2 ECD in patients treated with trastuzumab and paclitaxel, and among these patients, responses correlated with a decline in ECD levels over 12 weeks of therapy versus lower responses in those whose ECD levels remained high post-treatment [28].

A meta-analysis of eight clinical trials revealed that patients whose HER-2 ECD levels declined by at least 20% in the first few weeks after initiation of trastuzumab-based therapy had improved disease-free and overall survival compared with patients whose HER-2 ECD levels did not drop [29]. Hence, circulating ECD of HER-2 may be a serum marker useful for predicting response to trastuzumab. In contrast to these studies, a recent study by Anido and colleagues [30] suggests that truncated forms of HER-2 are actually the result of alternative initiation of translation from different methionines within the *her-2* sequence, which are referred to as C-terminal fragments of HER-2. The authors present compelling in vivo data showing that trastuzumab does not inhibit growth of mammary xenografts of the T47D breast cancer cell line stably transfected with the truncated form of HER-2, but does inhibit growth of T47D HER-2 stable transfectant xenografts. Hence, this study suggests that the presence of truncated forms of HER-2 may promote resistance to trastuzumab.

3.4 Amplification of Ligand-Induced Activation of ErbB Receptors

Exogenous ligands of the EGFR and HER3/4 co-receptors have been shown to rescue from the anti-proliferative effect of the antibody [31]. This is consistent with structural and cellular data using ErbB receptor ectodomains and different HER-2 monoclonal antibodies, which show that trastuzumab is unable to block ligand-induced EGFR/HER-2 and HER-2/HER3 heterodimers [32]. Recently, Ritter et al. [33] described a model of trastuzumab resistance by the generation of trastuzumab-resistant breast cancer cell line (BT-474) in vivo. The resistant cells retained HER-2 gene amplification and trastuzumab binding. They exhibited higher levels of phosphorylated EGFR (P-EGFR) and EGFR/ HER-2 heterodimers as well as over-expression of EGFR, transforming growth factor a (TGFa), heparin-binding EGF and heregulin RNAs compared with the parental, trastuzumab-sensitive cells, suggesting enhanced EGFR-mediated activation of HER-2. Small-molecule inhibitors of EGFR and HER-2 were effective against the antibody-resistant cells, suggesting that (a) they were still dependent on the ErbB receptor network and (b) amplification of ligand-induced activation of ErbB receptors is a potential mechanism of acquired resistance to trastuzumab.

4 IGF-IR Signalling Pathway in Breast Cancer

Similar to ErbB/HER family members, IGF-IR is a receptor tyrosine kinase that can be activated by binding to its ligands IGF-I and IGF-II and regulates the cell proliferation, survival and metastasis of cancer cells, including breast cancer cells. IGFBPs protect IGFs from degradation and negatively regulate the interaction between IGFs and their receptors [34]. Binding of IGFs to IGF-IR stimulates receptor tyrosine kinase and activate intracellular adaptor proteins, such as the insulin receptor substrate (IRS) family and SHC, MAPK and PI3K signalling pathway. Importantly, activation of PI3K/Akt signalling pathway subsequently stimulates mammalian target of rapamycin (mTOR), which results in mRNA translation and protein synthesis. Up-regulation of the IGF-IR signalling pathway increases the expression of cyclins and other proteins that are involved in maintaining cancer cell proliferation and survival. IGFs play an important role in maintaining the hallmarks of malignancy, including uncontrolled proliferation, survival and metastasis in breast cancer. IGF-IR activation affects motility and metastasis, and can also regulate the metastatic phenotype by enhancing invasion through the extracellular matrix, stimulating the secretion of matrix metalloproteinases, deregulating the expression or function of E-cadherin, and affecting cell migration and invasion. In addition, tissues expressing a higher level of IGFs, such as the lung and bone, are more frequent sites of breast cancer metastasis [35]. An increased IGF-IR signalling pathway has been found in breast cancers, and activation of IGF-IR signalling is well correlated with breast cancer progression, increased resistance to chemotherapy and radiotherapy, and indicative of a poor prognosis in breast cancer [36–38]. IGF-IR can interact with and activate HER-2 [39], and increased IGF-IR signalling has been associated with trastuzumab resistance [40]. Heterodimerisation between IGF-IR and HER-2 was observed in trastuzumab-resistant breast cancer cells and in gefitinib-resistant breast cancer cells [37, 38]. Esteva et al. previously reported that IGF-IR induces the phosphorylation of HER-2, which in turn is inhibited by the IGFIR tyrosine kinase inhibitor I-OMe-AG538 in trastuzumab-resistant breast cancer cells. They found IGF-IR and HER-2 heterodimerisation in trastuzumab-resistant cells but not in parental, trastuzumab-sensitive SKBR3 breast cancer cells. Importantly, anti-IGF-IR agents restored trastuzumab sensitivity and decreased cell viability in trastuzumab-resistant cells [38]. Similarly, HER-2 blockade also disrupted heterodimerisation and inhibited cell viability in trastuzumab-resistant cells. These results suggest that targeting IGF-IR might be a useful strategy in trastuzumab-resistant breast cancers in which heterodimerisation and signal crosstalk exist between IGF-IR and HER-2. Interestingly, IGFBP3, which blocks IGF1-mediated activation of IGF-IR, has been shown to arrest growth in trastuzumab-resistant cells. Other investigators have further explored the ability of IGFBP3 to suppress HER-2-over-expressing breast tumour growth and restore the tumours' sensitivity to trastuzumab [41]. Treatment with recombinant human IGFBP3 (rhIGFBP3) has shown significant dose-dependent growth inhibition of trastuzumab-resistant HER-2-over-expressing breast cancer cells with increased IGF-IR levels and enhanced the antitumour effect of trastuzumab in vitro and in vivo, due to the ability of rhIGFBP3 to inhibit HER-2- and IGF-IR-mediated activation of the Ras/MAPK and PI3K/Akt pathways. Thus, combining HER-2 and IGF-IR targeting agents might be an effective therapeutic strategy for trastuzumab-resistant HER-2-over-expressing breast cancer.

Decreased p27Kip1 expression has been observed in trastuzumab-resistant cells derived from the SKBR3 cell line [42], and inhibition of p27Kip1 expression levels by small interfering RNA resulted in decreased sensitivity to trastuzumab in HER-2-over-expressing SKBR3 breast cancer cells [43]. Trastuzumab sensitivity in the cells was restored by increasing the expression of exogenous p27Kip1 via transfection or of endogenous p27Kip1 by the proteasome inhibitor MG132. These results indicate that p27Kip1 plays a critical role in the response to trastuzumab and that it might be useful as a therapeutic target in trastuzumab-resistant breast cancers [42]. The decrease in p27Kip1 protein levels in trastuzumab-resistant cells is possibly regulated by upstream signalling of p27Kip1, such as the crosstalk between HER-2 and IGF-IR, leading to the activation of the IGF-IR-mediated PI3K/Akt signal pathway, resulting in p27Kip1 degradation by ubiquitin ligase SKP2 and contributing to trastuzumab resistance [38]. The protein level of p27Kip1 was also decreased in response to IGF-I in parental and resistant SKBR3 cells. Thus, trastuzumab resistance mediated by p27Kip1 could be overcome by targeting IGF-IR signalling by either antibody blockade or kinase inhibition, demonstrating the potential importance of IGF-IR signalling pathway as a therapeutic target in trastuzumab-resistant breast cancer.

5 Conclusions

The increasing evidence of trastuzumab resistance in breast cancer patients is becoming very important, considering also the use of this drug in the adjuvant setting. Therefore understanding the mechanisms of non-response to trastuzumab is urgently needed to provide alternative strategies to overcome resistance.

References

1. Hynes NE, Lane HA (2005) ERBB receptors and cancer: the complexity of targeted inhibitors. Nat Rev Cancer 5:341–354
2. Ramsauer VP, Carraway CA, Salas PJ, Carraway KL (2003) Muc4/ sialomucin complex, the intramembrane ErbB2 ligand, translocates ErbB2 to the apical surface in polarized epithelial cells. J Biol Chem 278:30142–30147
3. Holbro T, Beerli RR, Maurer F, Koziczak M, Barbas CF 3rd, Hynes NE (2003) The ErbB2/ ErbB3 heterodimer functions as an oncogenic unit: ErbB2 requires ErbB3 to drive breast tumor cell proliferation. Proc Natl Acad Sci USA 100:8933–8938
4. Wang SC, Lien HC, Xia W, Chen IF, Lo HW, Wang Z, Ali-Seyed M, Lee DF, Bartholomeusz G, Ou-Yang F et al (2004) Binding at and transactivation of the COX-2 promoter by nuclear tyrosine kinase receptor ErbB-2. Cancer Cell 6:251–261
5. Klijn JG, Berns PM, Schmitz PI, Foekens JA (1992) The clinical significance of epidermal growth factor receptor (EGF-R) in human breast cancer: a review on 5232 patients. Endocr Rev 13:3–17
6. Perou CM, Sorlie T, Eisen MB, van de Rijn M, Jeffrey SS, Rees CA, Pollack JR, Ross DT, Johnsen H, Akslen LA et al (2000) Molecular portraits of human breast tumours. Nature 406:747–752
7. Owens MA, Horten BC, Da Silva MM (2004) HER2 amplification ratios by fluorescence in situ hybridization and correlation with immunohistochemistry in a cohort of 6556 breast cancer tissues. Clin Breast Cancer 5:63–69
8. Romond EH, Perez EA, Bryant J, Suman VJ, Geyer CE Jr, Davidson NE, Tan-Chiu E, Martino S, Paik S, Kaufman PA et al (2005) Trastuzumab plus adjuvant chemotherapy for operable HER2-positive breast cancer. N Engl J Med 353:1673–1684
9. Piccart-Gebhart MJ, Procter M, Leyland-Jones B, Goldhirsch A, Untch M, Smith I, Gianni L, Baselga J, Bell R, Jackisch C et al (2005) Trastuzumab after adjuvant chemotherapy in HER2-positive breast cancer. N Engl J Med 353:1659–1672
10. Buzdar AU, Ibrahim NK, Francis D, Booser DJ, Thomas ES, Theriault RL, Pusztai L, Green MC, Arun BK, Giordano SH et al (2005) Significantly higher pathologic complete remission rate after neoadjuvant therapy with trastuzumab, paclitaxel, and epirubicin chemotherapy: results of a randomized trial in human epidermal growth factor receptor 2-positive operable breast cancer. J Clin Oncol 23:3676–3685
11. Nahta R, Esteva FJ (2006) Herceptin: mechanisms of action and resistance. Cancer Lett 232:123–138
12. Nagata Y, Lan KH, Zhou X, Tan M, Esteva FJ, Sahin AA, Klos KS, Li P, Monia BP, Nguyen NT et al (2004) PTEN activation contributes to tumor inhibition by trastuzumab, and loss of PTEN predicts trastuzumab resistance in patients. Cancer Cell 6:117–127
13. Cooley S, Burns LJ, Repka T, Miller JS (1999) Natural killer cell cytotoxicity of breast cancer targets is enhanced by two distinct mechanisms of antibody-dependent cellular cytotoxicity against LFA-3 and HER2/neu. Exp Hematol 27:1533–1541

14. Izumi Y, Xu L, di Tomaso E, Fukumura D, Jain RK (2002) Tumour biology: Herceptin acts as an anti-angiogenic cocktail. Nature 416:279–280
15. Klos KS, Zhou X, Lee S, Zhang L, Yang W, Nagata Y, Yu D (2003) Combined trastuzumab and paclitaxel treatment better inhibits ErbB-2-mediated angiogenesis in breast carcinoma through a more effective inhibition of Akt than either treatment alone. Cancer 98:1377–1385
16. Baselga J, Tripathy D, Mendelsohn J, Baughman S, Benz CC, Dantis L, Sklarin NT, Seidman AD, Hudis CA, Moore J et al (1996) Phase II study of weekly intravenous recombinant humanized anti-p185HER2 monoclonal antibody in patients with HER2/neu-overexpressing metastatic breast cancer. J Clin Oncol 14:737–744
17. Seidman AD, Fornier MN, Esteva FJ, Tan L, Kaptain S, Bach A, Panageas KS, Arroyo C, Valero V, Currie V et al (2001) Weekly trastuzumab and paclitaxel therapy for metastatic breast cancer with analysis of efficacy by HER2 immunophenotype and gene amplification. J Clin Oncol 19:2587–2595
18. Slamon DJ, Leyland-Jones B, Shak S, Fuchs H, Paton V, Bajamonde A, Fleming T, Eiermann W, Wolter J, Pegram M et al (2001) Use of chemotherapy plus a monoclonal antibody against HER2 for metastatic breast cancer that overexpresses HER2. N Engl J Med 344:783–792
19. Esteva FJ, Valero V, Booser D, Guerra LT, Murray JL, Pusztai L, Cristofanilli M, Arun B, Esmaeli B, Fritsche HA et al (2002) Phase II study of weekly docetaxel and trastuzumab for patients with HER-2-overexpressing metastatic breast cancer. J Clin Oncol 20:1800–1808
20. Nahta R, Yu D, Hung MC, Hortobagyi GN, Esteva FJ (2006) Mechanisms of disease: understanding resistance to HER2-targeted therapy in human breast cancer. Nat Clin Pract Oncol 3:269–280
21. Price-Schiavi SA, Jepson S, Li P, Arango M, Rudland PS, Yee L, Carraway KL (2002) Rat Muc4 (sialomucin complex) reduces binding of anti-ErbB2 antibodies to tumor cell surfaces, a potential mechanism for herceptin resistance. Int J Cancer 99:783–791
22. Nagy P, Friedlander E, Tanner M, Kapanen AI, Carraway KL, Isola J, Jovin TM (2005) Decreased accessibility and lack of activation of ErbB2 in JIMT-1, a herceptin-resistant, MUC4-expressing breast cancer cell line. Cancer Res 65:473–482
23. Carraway KL, Price-Schiavi SA, Komatsu M, Jepson S, Perez A, Carraway CA (2001) Muc4/sialomucin complex in the mammary gland and breast cancer. J Mammary Gland Biol Neoplasia 6:323–337
24. Yakes FM, Chinratanalab W, Ritter CA, King W, Seelig S, Arteaga CL (2002) Herceptin-induced inhibition of phosphatidylinositol- 3 kinase and Akt is required for antibody-mediated effects on p27, cyclin D1, and antitumor action. Cancer Res 62:4132–4141
25. Chan CT, Metz MZ, Kane SE (2005) Differential sensitivities of trastuzumab (Herceptin)-resistant human breast cancer cells to phosphoinositide-3 kinase (PI-3K) and epidermal growth factor receptor (EGFR) kinase inhibitors. Breast Cancer Res Treat 91:187–201
26. Lin YZ, Clinton GM (1991) A soluble protein related to the HER-2 proto-oncogene product is released from human breast carcinoma cells. Oncogene 6:639–643
27. Yamauchi H, O'Neill A, Gelman R, Carney W, Tenney DY, Hosch S, Hayes DF (1997) Prediction of response to antiestrogen therapy in advanced breast cancer patients by pretreatment circulating levels of extracellular domain of the HER-2/c-neu protein. J Clin Oncol 15:2518–2525
28. Fornier MN, Seidman AD, Schwartz MK, Ghani F, Thiel R, Norton L, Hudis C (2005) Serum HER2 extracellular domain in metastatic breast cancer patients treated with weekly trastuzumab and paclitaxel: association with HER2 status by immunohistochemistry and fluorescence in situ hybridization and with response rate. Ann Oncol 16:234–239
29. Ali SM, Esteva FJ, Fornier M, Gligorov J, Harris L, Kostler WJ, Luftner D, Pichon MF, Tse C, Lipton A (2006) Serum HER-2/neu change predicts clinical outcome to trastuzumab-based therapy. J Clin Oncol 24(Suppl):500
30. Anido J, Scaltriti M, Bech Serra JJ, Santiago Josefat B, Todo FR, Baselga J, Arribas J (2006) Biosynthesis of tumorigenic HER2 C-terminal fragments by alternative initiation of translation. EMBO J 25:3234–3244

31. Motoyama AB, Hynes NE, Lane HA (2002) The efficacy of ErbB receptor-targeted anticancer therapeutics is influenced byt he availability of epidermal growth factor-related peptides. Cancer Res 62:3151–3158
32. Agus DB, Akita RW, Fox WD, Lewis GD, Higgins B, Pisacane PI, Lofgren JA, Tindell C, Evans DP, Maiese K et al (2002) Targeting ligand activated ErbB2 signaling inhibits breast and prostate tumor growth. Cancer Cell 2:127–137
33. Ritter CA, Perez-Torres M, Rinehart C, Guix M, Dugger T, Engelman JA, Arteaga CL (2007) Human breast cancer cells selected for resistance to rastuzumab in vivo overexpress epidermal growth factor receptor and ErbB ligands and remain dependent on the ErbB receptor network. Clin Cancer Res 13:4909–4919
34. Firth SM, Baxter RC (2002) Cellular actions of the insulin-like growth factor binding proteins. Endocr Rev 23:824–854
35. Sangai T, Fujimoto H, Miyamoto S, Maeda H, Nakamura M, Ishii G, Nagai K, Nagashima T, Miyazaki M, Ochiai A et al (2008) Roles of osteoclasts and bone-derived IGFs in the survival and growth of human breast cancer cells in human adult bone implanted into nonobese diabetic/severe combined immunodeficient mice. Clin Exp Metastasis 25:401–410
36. Morgillo F, Woo JK, Kim ES, Hong WK, Lee HY (2006) Heterodimerization of insulin-like growth factor receptor/epidermal growth factor receptor and induction of survivin expression counteract the antitumor action of erlotinib. Cancer Res 66:10100–10111
37. Jones HE, Goddard L, Gee JM, Hiscox S, Rubini M, Barrow D, Knowlden JM, Williams S, Wakeling AE, Nicholson RI et al (2004). Insulin-like growth factor-I receptor signalling and acquired resistance to gefitinib (ZD1839; Iressa) in human breast and prostate cancer cells. Endocr Relat Cancer 11:793–814
38. Nahta R, Yuan LX, Zhang B, Kobayashi R, Esteva FJ (2005) Insulin like growth factor-I receptor/human epidermal growth factor receptor 2 heterodimerization contributes to trastuzumab resi stance of breast cancer cells. Cancer Res 65:11118–11128
39. Balana ME, Labriola L, Salatino M, Movsichoff F, Peters G, Charreau EH, Elizalde PV (2001) Activation of ErbB-2 via a hierarchical interaction between ErbB-2 and type I insulin-like growth factor receptor in mammary tumor cells. Oncogene 20:34–47
40. Lu Y, Zi X, Zhao Y, Mascarenhas D, Pollak M (2001) Insulin-like growth factor-I receptor signaling and resistance to trastuzumab (Herceptin). J Natl Cancer Inst 93:1852–1857
41. Jerome L, Alami N, Belanger S, Page V, Yu Q, Paterson J, Shiry L, Pegram M, Leyland-Jones B (2006) Recombinant human insulin-like growth factor binding protein 3 inhibits growth of human epidermal growth factor receptor-2- overexpressing breast tumors and potentiates herceptin activity in vivo. Cancer Res 66:7245–7252
42. Nahta R, Hung MC, Esteva FJ (2004) The HER-2-targeting antibodies trastuzumab and pertuzumab synergistically inhibit the survival of breast cancer cells. Cancer Res 4:2343–2346
43. Le XF, Claret FX, Lammayot A, Tian L, Deshpande D, LaPushin R, Tari AM, Bast RC Jr (2003) The role of cyclin-dependent kinase inhibitor p27Kip1 in anti-HER2 antibody-induced G1 cell cycle arrest and tumor growth inhibition. J Biol Chem 278:23441–23450

Treatment with Trastuzumab Beyond Progression

Gunter von Minckwitz and Cristina Pirvulescu

Abstract Trastuzumab is the first antibody that has shown clinical activity in patients with HER-2-positive breast cancer. The mechanism of action is not fully understood; however, antibody-derived cellular cytotoxicity (ADCC) is considered to explain important peculiarities of its clinical activity such as treatment beyond progression. Based on early pre-clinical data, trastuzumab was used beyond progression since the start of its clinical use. Initially evidence to use trastuzumab beyond progression came only from observational studies, which might have been biased by the unknown decision criteria for or against continuation of trastuzumab. Only recently, the randomised GBG 26 study demonstrated that capecitabine and continuing trastuzumab beyond progression achieved a higher response rate and longer progression-free survival than capecitabine alone. Supportive evidence came from studies combining trastuzumab with lapatinib or pertuzumab in trastuzumab pre-treated patients, showing better results than the same treatment without trastuzumab. A blockade of HER-2 throughout all stages of Her-2-positive breast cancer should therefore be considered.

1 Introduction

Therapeutic strategies have been developed in order to block the HER-2 signalling pathways, and to improve the outcome of patients. With the development of trastuzumab, a new clinically relevant subgroup of breast cancer was established [1]. Especially in combination with cytotoxic agents, not only very promising

G. von Minckwitz (✉)
German Breast Group, c/o GBG Forschungs GmbH, Martin-Behaim Str. 12, 63263 Neu-Isenburg/Frankfurt am Main, Germany
e-mail: gunter.vonminckwitz@germanbreastgroup.de

M. Sibilia et al. (eds.), *Drugs for HER-2-positive Breast Cancer*,
Milestones in Drug Therapy, DOI 10.1007/978-3-0346-0094-1_4,

response rates but also an improvement in survival could be demonstrated for treatment with trastuzumab [2, 3]. Patients with HER-2-positive metastatic breast cancer treated repeatedly with trastuzumab at the MD Anderson Hospital, Houston, have demonstrated a 2-year overall survival better than patients with HER-2-negative disease. With this targeted agent in hand, positive HER-2 status cannot be considered any longer as a negative but rather as a positive prognostic factor [4].

However, despite very long periods of disease control, most patients with HER-2-positive MBC develop resistance to trastuzumab [5, 6].

Change of treatment at disease progression is a general principle in oncology. It is not known whether this holds true for novel biological agents such as trastuzumab. Reports on effects of trastuzumab beyond progression were made from the very beginning of the clinical use of this drug. Increasing evidence from preclinical data, retrospective cohort, phase II and phase III studies now supports this concept, which represents a paradigm shift of treatment pattern in oncology.

2 Mechanisms of Action of Trastuzumab

Four main mechanisms are currently under discussion to explain clinical activity to trastuzumab.

Trastuzumab blocks HER-2 activated cell proliferation [7]. HER-2 signalling initiates cell proliferation, differentiation and survival. In tumour cells with over-expression of HER-2 increased signalling leads to increased cell proliferation. Trastuzumab blocks the activation of HER-2 signalling and reduces cell proliferation.

Trastuzumab prevents the formation of $p95^{HER\text{-}2}$ [8]. $P95^{HER\text{-}2}$ is a highly active, truncated isoform of HER-2, where the extracellular domain is cleaved by metalloproteinases. When trastuzumab is bound to the extracellular domain, metalloproteinases cannot cleave this domain and down-stream signalling is prevented.

Activated HER-2 is also involved in inducing tumour neo-angiogenesis [9]. By inhibition of HER-2, trastuzumab also decreases neo-angiogenesis and therefore the blood supply to the tumour.

Trastuzumab mediates the antibody-dependent cellular cytotoxicity (ADCC) and activates the body's own immune response [10]. When trastuzumab binds to HER-2, natural killer cells are recruited that can bind via their Fcγ-receptor to the Fc domain of the antibody. Thus activated, the natural killer cells release cytolytic agents and destroy the tumour cells. Polymorphisms of the Fcγ-receptor are currently investigated as modulators of trastuzumab activity [11].

Especially the last mechanism could be an explanation for maintaining activity of trastuzumab throughout the course of metastatic disease.

3 Preclinical Evidence for Treatment Beyond Progression with Trastuzumab

The rule to stop treatment at disease progression derives from the traditional clinical management of cytotoxic agents. Cumulative toxicity did not allow continuation of the use of these agents as long as no proof for restoration of efficacy was available. The switch to ideally non-cross resistant agents was the preferred way in general.

It has been argued, however, that this paradigm may not apply to molecularly targeted drugs such as trastuzumab. Preclinical data indicate that trastuzumab is effective against tumour cell proliferation as long as it is present, whereas trastuzumab withdrawal results in rapid tumour cell re-growth [12, 13]. Tripathy and colleagues found out that breast cancer cell proliferation is inhibited partially by continuing trastuzumab even after the development of resistance [14]. Furthermore, trastuzumab significantly enhances the anti-tumour effect of taxanes in tumours progressing under trastuzumab alone [15]. Conversely, Nahta and colleagues report that the continuation of trastuzumab beyond development of resistance did not improve the efficacy of chemotherapy, e.g. vinorelbine [16]. As these investigations are best on cell line experiments, they cannot account for the activity of trastuzumab mediated by ADCC. Barok et al. could demonstrate in an in-vivo model that trastuzumab was active not only in a sensitive transplanted breast cancer cell line, but also in an in vitro trastuzumab-resistant cell line [17]. So, it appears that activity of trastuzumab cannot sufficiently be predicted by in-vitro experiments, in-vivo experiments might be preferable, but finally clinical activity beyond progression remains to be demonstrated.

4 Evidence from Retrospective Cohort and Phase II Studies Supporting Treatment Beyond Progression with Trastuzumab

Clinical evidence on treatment with trastuzumab beyond progression with a switch to a different chemotherapy was reported from various retrospective analyses (Table 1). The largest prospective study [19] was a non-randomised extension study to the pivotal phase III trial (H0648g)[2], where patients progressing after first-line chemotherapy and trastuzumab switched to another chemotherapy and continued trastuzumab. The objective response rate was modest with 11% and the duration of response was 6 months. Other prospective, non-randomised studies reported response rates of 18–29% and a time to progression of 8.0 months however, the sample sizes were small including a maximum of 40 patients per trial. Several retrospective observational cohort studies reported response rates of up to 50% [21, 22, 32] however, these results might be biased due to unknown factors influencing physicians' decision to stop or to continue trastuzumab. As an example, a large observational study assessed 910 patients treated with trastuzumab

Table 1 Overview of observational and phase II trastuzumab treatment beyond progression studies

Study	*N* (Second line Trastuzumab)	Study cohort	Response to Second trastuzumab containing regimes	
			ORR (%)	TTP (months)
Fountzilas et al. (2003) [18]	80	Mono-institutional, retrospective analysis 80 HER-2 over-expressed MBC (IHC 2+ or 3+)	24	5.2
Tripathy et al. (2004) [19]	93	Extension study to a pivotal phase III trial (H0648g) 120 HER-2 over-expressed MBC (IHC 3+)	11	n.r.
Gelmon et al. (2004) [20]	65	Multi-institutional, retrospective analysis 105 HER-2 over-expressed MBC (IHC 2+ or 3+)	32	6.0
García-Sáenz et al. (2005) [21]	31	Mono-institutional, retrospective analysis 58 HER-2 over-expressed MBC (IHC 2+ or 3+)	26	3.0
Stemmler et al. (2005) [22]	23	Retrospective analysis 136 HER-2 over expressed MBC (IHC 3+)	39	6.0
Tokajuk et al. (2006) [23]	14	Retrospective analysis 27 HER-2 over-expressed MBC (IHC 3+)	50	5.1
Morabito et al. (2006) [24]	26	Phase II, monocentric, one arm study (trastuzumab+ gemcitabine+vinorelbine) 26 HER-2 over-expressed MBC (IHC 2+ or 3+)	29	n.r.
Bartsch et al. (2006) [25]	54	Prospective, observational study 54 HER-2 over expressed MBC (IHC 3+, FISH)	26	6.0
Montemurro et al. (2006) [26]	40	Retrospective analysis 132 HER-2 over-expressed MBC (IHC 3+)	18	6.3
Orlando et al. (2006) [27]	22	Prospective, one arm, observational study (metronomic CM+ trastuzumab) 22 HER-2 over-expressed MBC (IHC 3+, FISH)	18	6.0
Bachelot et al. (2007) [28]	17	Phase II, multicenter, 2-step trial (vinorelbine+trastuzumab) 17 HER-2 over-expressed MBC (IHC 3+, FISH, CISH)	29	n.r.
Bartsch et al. (2007) [29]	40	Prospective, monocentric, one arm study (capecitabine+trastuzumab)	20	8.0

(*continued*)

Table 1 (continued)

Study	*N* (Second line Trastuzumab)	Study cohort	Response to Second trastuzumab containing regimes	
			ORR (%)	TTP (months)
		40 HER-2 over-expressed MBC (IHC 3+, FISH)		
Metro et al. (2007) [30]	37	Retrospective analysis 69 HER-2 over-expressed MBC	29	6.7
Jackisch et al. (2007) [31]	112	Retrospective observational study 112 HER-2 over-expressed MBC with continued trastuzumab treatment (compared with 81 patients which discontinued trastuzumab treatment)	n.r.	20.1 (vs. 13.4 for patients without trastuzumab)

n.r. not reported

for metastatic disease in Germany [31]. Treatment of trastuzumab beyond progression was recorded in 112 patients, where with 81 patients showed tumour progression and were treated with another chemotherapy without trastuzumab. Baseline demographics and prior therapy were similar in the two treatment groups. However, overall survival was significantly increased in patients continuing trastuzumab treatment beyond disease progression (time to subsequent progression: 20.1 vs. 13.4 months).

5 Phase III Evidence Supporting the Concept of Treatment Beyond Progression with Trastuzumab

Initial attempts in the USA (MD Anderson Cancer Centre and South West Oncology Group) to investigate trastuzumab beyond progression in combination with vinorelbine in prospective randomised trials have failed because a strong prevision by physicians and patients for the superiority of this continuation approach resulted in insufficient accrual.

The first evidence came from a randomised trial comparing lapatinib in combination with capecitabine vs. capecitabine alone in patients previously treated with trastuzumab [33, 34]. Lapatinib increased the efficacy of capecitabine by improving the response rate from 14.3% to 22.5% and prolonging time to progression from 4.3 to 6.2 months. These results can of course be explained by not only a non-cross resistance of the two anti-HER-2 agents, but also by a general synergism of both anti-HER-2 treatments in combination with cytotoxic agents even beyond progression.

6 The GBG 26 Treatment Beyond Progression Study

The GBG 26 TBP trial [35] was conducted by the German Breast Group together with groups from Austria, Denmark, Netherlands, Slovenia and the UK and provides now the only phase III evidence for continuing trastuzumab beyond progression in patients with HER-2-positive MBC. Capecitabine monotherapy was chosen as chemotherapy as it was the only agent approved by the authorities for the treatment of patients with MBC resistance to both anthracycline and paclitaxel. Capecitabine produces objective response rates of 20–25% with a median duration of 5 months in this patient population. The combination of capecitabine and trastuzumab showed a clinical benefit rate of 63–70% in heavily pre-treated patients with HER-2-positive advanced breast cancer [36]. The initial plan was to recruit 482 patients to demonstrate an improvement of 27.5% in the time to progression (4.0 months with capecitabine alone and 5.1 months with capecitabine and continued trastuzumab). Despite over 50 actively participating sites, accrual was very slow, so that the trial was closed after randomisation of 156 patients, when the lapatinib became registered in this setting.

Seventy-eight patients were randomised to capecitabine alone (X; 2,500 mg/m^2 on days 1–14, q21), and 78 to capecitabine plus continuation of trastuzumab (XH; 6 mg/kg, q3w) (Fig. 1). Patients were randomised and stratified according to pre-treatment: taxanes/trastuzumab as first-line therapy ($n = 111$), taxanes/trastuzumab as adjuvant therapy ($n = 3$), and trastuzumab alone or without taxanes as first-line treatment ($n = 42$). Half of the patients were also pre-treated with anthracyclines. After a median follow-up of 15.6 months, the median time to progression was 5.6 months in the capecitabine group and 8.2 months in the capecitabine plus trastuzumab group with an unadjusted hazard ratio of 0.69 (95% confidence interval [95% CI]: 0.48–0.97; 2-sided log-rank test $P = 0.0338$). Overall response rates were 27.0% with capecitabine and 48.1% with capecitabine plus trastuzumab (odds

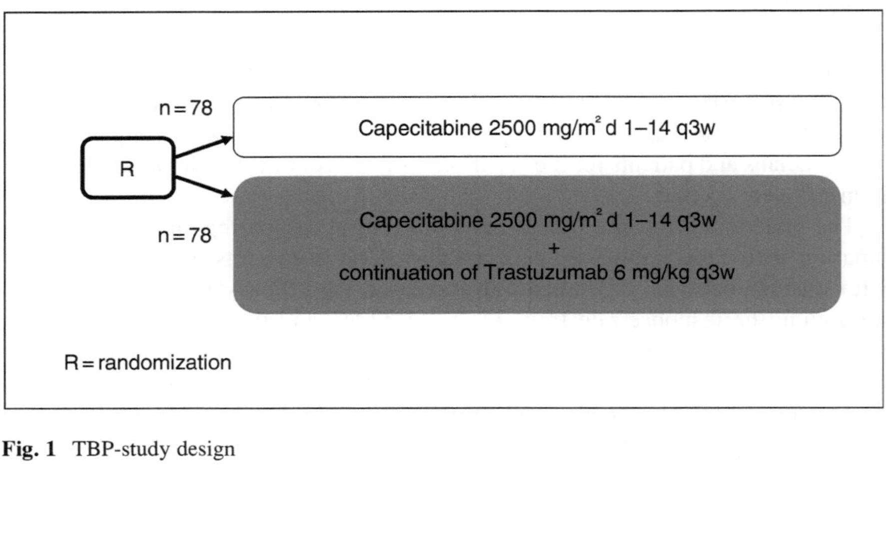

Fig. 1 TBP-study design

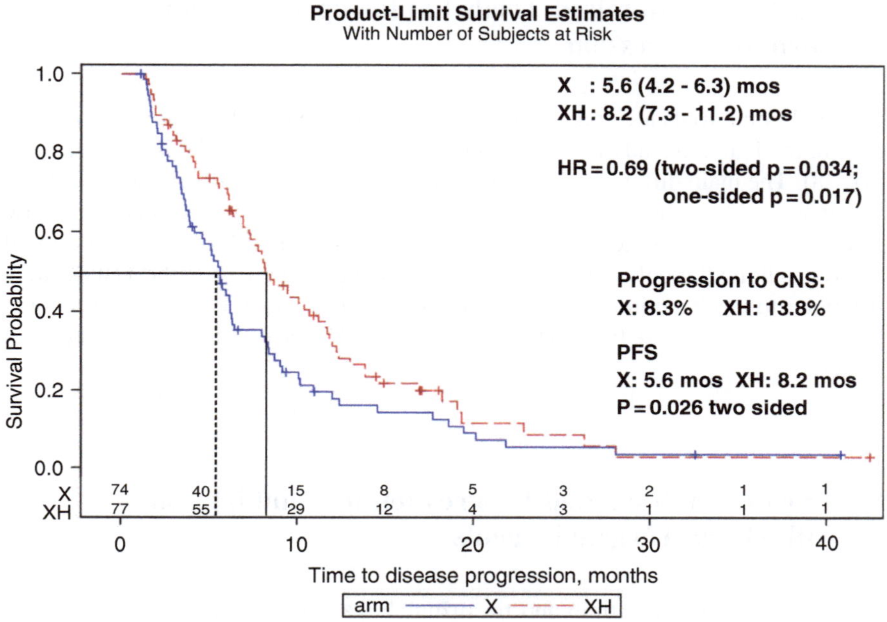

Fig. 2 Time to progression, primary end point of the GBG 26 TBP study comparing capecitabine (X) with X and continued trastuzumab beyond progression (XH) [35]

ratio = 2.50; $P = 0.0115$). Brain metastases were also observed in this trial in eight patients receiving the combination therapy, and in five patients treated with X alone (Fig. 2).

Continuing trastuzumab beyond progression was not associated with an increase in toxicity. The incidence of cardiac morbidities was low in both arms (2.7% with X and 5.2% with XH, but only one patient with a decrease in left ventricular ejection fraction of below 40%). It has to be considered that the median time on trastuzumab treatment before entering the study was 45 weeks and cardiac co-morbidities was an exclusion criterion, so that most patients at risk for trastuzumab-induced cardiac toxicity were excluded from trial participation.

Overall survival was 20.4 (95% CI: 17.8–24.7) months in the capecitabine group and 25.5 (95% CI: 19.0–30.7) months in the capecitabine plus trastuzumab group ($P = 0.257$). Long-term follow-up data will be available at the end of 2010.

The GBG 26 trial has several strengths and limitations. The results consistently show superior efficacy of continuation of trastuzumab in the adjusted and sensitivity analyses. The trial investigated in a straightforward prospective way the beyond progression approach as all patients progressed during trastuzumab. Patients in the capecitabine group probably had an ongoing exposure to trastuzumab due its long half-life. Due to premature closure of the trial, the number of patients included in the trial is small, but it is the only trial worldwide that reached a sufficient sample size for statistical analysis.

7 Further Randomised Trials Exploring Treatment Beyond Progression

Two additional trials are conducted in Europe and in only Italy with a comparable design; the Pandora study and the THOR (Trastuzumab Halted Or Retained) study [37, 38]. The main difference in designs of these two trials compared with GBG 26 is that second line chemotherapy was not fixed, but the investigators could choose among numerous regimens enlisted in the protocols. The Pandora study closed randomisation after only about 20 patients due to poor accrual and the THOR study still plans to reach a minimum target accrual of 80 patients. It is planned to conduct a meta-analysis of these two trials together with GBG 26 to achieve more statistical power.

8 Trastuzumab Beyond Progression in Combination with Other Targeted Agents

The combination of lapatinib and trastuzumab was investigated in a large randomised phase II study including 296 heavily and trastuzumab pre-treated patients with HER-2-positive metastatic breast cancer [39]. As the control arm was lapatinib therapy alone, this design also represents a treatment beyond progression trial. The continuation of trastuzumab prolonged the time to progression from 8.1 to 12.0 weeks (HR 0.73; $p = 0.008$) in this unfavourable group of patients.

An interesting result was also reported for the combination of trastuzumab with pertuzumab, an antibody directed against the dimerisation epitope of the HER-2 receptor that inhibits the dimerisation of HER-2 with other HER family receptors. This phase II study reported on 66 patients all pre-treated with trastuzumab [40]. The combination of both agents resulted in an objective response rate of 24.2% and a clinical benefit rate of 50.0%. As pertuzumab alone in another trial did not show any clinical activity in a comparable setting, also these results have to be explained by the activity of trastuzumab beyond progression.

9 Conclusion and Future Perspectives

There is growing evidence in the literature for the use of trastuzumab beyond disease progression. Antibody-derived cellular cytotoxicity (ADCC) might be the relevant mechanism for this so far, not for other treatment observed concept. It is supported by various in-vivo data and evidence from multiple cohort study as well as by a randomised phase III study not only for the combination with chemotherapy, but also for the combination with other anti-HER-2 agents.

To further improve the prognosis of patients with HER-2-positive metastatic breast cancer even beyond that of patients with HER-2-negative disease, a blockade of HER-2 throughout all stages of early and metastatic breast cancer should be considered.

References

1. Chazin VR, Kaleko M, Miller AD, Slamon DJ (1992) Transformation mediated by the human HER2neu gene independent of the epidermal growth factor receptor. Oncogene 7:1859–1866
2. Slamon DJ, Leyland-Jones B, Shak S et al (2001) Use of chemotherapy plus a monoclonal antibody against HER2 for metastatic breast cancer that overexpresses HER2. N Engl J Med 344:783–792
3. Giordano S, Buzdar A, Smith T, Kau SW, Yang Y, Hortobabgy G (2004) Is breast cancer survival improving? trends in survival for patients with recurrent breast cancer diagnosed from 1974 through 2000. Cancer 100(199):44–52
4. Dawood SS, Kristine B, Hortobagyi GN, Giordiano SH (2008) Prognosis of women with stage IV breast cancer by HER2 status and trastuzumab treatment: an institutional based review. J Clin Oncol 26(Suppl): abstract 1018
5. Romond EH, Perez EA, Bryant J et al (2005) Trastuzumab plus adjuvant chemotherapy for operable HER2-positive breast cancer. N Engl J Med 353:1673–1684
6. Piccart-Gebhart MJ, Procter M, Leyland-Jones B et al (2005) Trastuzumab after adjuvant chemotherapy in HER2-positive breast cancer. N Engl J Med 353:1659–1672
7. Nahta R, Esteva FJ (2006) HER2 therapy: molecular mechanisms of trastuzumab resistance. Breast Cancer Res 8(6):215
8. Molina MA, Codony-Servat J, Albanell J, Rojo F, Arribas J, Baselga J (2001) Trastuzumab (herceptin), a humanized anti-Her2 receptor monoclonal antibody, inhibits basal and activated Her2 ectodomain cleavage in breast cancer cells. Cancer Res 61:4744–4749
9. Izumi Y, Xu L, di Tomaso E, Fukumura D, Jain RK (2002) Tumour biology: herceptin acts as an anti-angiogenic cocktail. Nature 416:279–280
10. Clynes RA, Towers TL, Presta LG, Ravetch JV (2000) Inhibitory Fc receptors modulate in vivo cytoxicity against tumor targets. Nat Med 6(4):443–446
11. Musolino A, Naldi N, Bortesi B, Pezzuolo D, Capelletti M, Missale G et al (2008) Immunoglobulin G fragment C receptor polymorphisms and clinical efficacy of trastuzumab-based therapy in patients with HER-2/neu-positive metastatic breast cancer. J Clin Oncol 26:1789–1796
12. Pegram MD, Konecny GE, O'Callaghan C, Beryt M, Pietras R, Slamon DJ (2004) Rational combinations of trastuzumab with chemotherapeutic drugs used in the treatment of breast cancer. J Natl Cancer Inst 96(10):739–749
13. Pietras RJ, Pegram MD, Finn RS, Maneval DA, Slamon DJ (1998) Remission of human breast cancer xenografts on therapy with humanized monoclonal antibody to HER-2 receptor and DNA-reactive drugs. Oncogene 17(17):2235–2249
14. Tripathy D, Hassan S, Verma S, Gurnani P, Nandi A, Rosenblatt K (2005) Phenotypic and proteomic alterations of acquired trastuzumab resistance. J Clin Oncol 23(suppl):3121
15. Bullock K, Blackwell K (2008) Clinical efficacy of taxane-trastuzumab combination regimens for HER-2-positive metastatic breast cancer. Oncologist 13(5):515–525
16. Nahta R, Esteva FJ (2004) In vitro effects of trastuzumab and vinorelbine in trastuzumab-resistant breast cancer cells. Cancer Chemother Pharmacol 53:186–190
17. Barok M, Isola J, Pályi-Krekk Z, Nagy P, Juhász I, Vereb G et al (2007) Trastuzumab causes antibody-dependent cellular cytotoxicity-mediated growth inhibition of submacroscopic

JIMT-1 breast cancer xenografts despite intrinsic drug resistance. J Mol Cancer Ther 6:2065–2072
18. Fountzilas G, Razis E, Tsavdaridis D, Karina M, Labropoulos S, Christodoulou C, Mavroudis D, Gogas H, Georgoulias V, Skarlos D (2003) Continuation of trastuzumab beyond disease progression is feasible and safe in patients with metastatic breast cancer: a retrospective analysis of 80 cases by the hellenic cooperative oncology group. Clin Breast Cancer 4 (2):120–125
19. Tripathy D, Slamon DJ, Cobleigh M, Arnold A, Saleh M, Mortimer JE, Murphy M, Stewart SJ (2004) Safety of treatment of metastatic breast cancer with trastuzumab beyond disease progression. J Clin Oncol 22(6):1063–1070
20. Gelmon KA, Mackey J, Verma S, Gertler SZ, Bangemann N, Klimo P, Schneeweiss A, Bremer K, Soulieres D, Tonkin K, Bell R, Heinrich B, Grenier D, Dias R (2004) Use of trastuzumab beyond disease progression: observations from a retrospective review of case histories. Clin Breast Cancer 5(1):52–58; discussion 59–62
21. García-Sáenz JA, Martín M, Puente J et al (2005) Trastuzumab associated with successive cytotoxic therapies beyond disease progression in metastatic breast cancer. Clin Breast Cancer 6:325–329
22. Stemmler HJ, Kahlert S, Siekiera W et al (2005) Prolonged survival of patients receiving trastuzumab beyond disease progression for HER2 overexpressing metastatic breast cancer (MBC). Onkologie 28:582–586
23. Tokajuk P, Czartoryska-Arlukowicz B, Wojtukiewicz MZ (2006) Activity of trastuzumab-based therapy beyond disease progression in heavily pretreated metastatic breast cancer patients – single institution experience. ASCO Annual Meeting Proceedings Part I. J Clin Oncol 24(18S):13159
24. Morabito A, Longo R, Gattuso D, Carillio G, Massaccesi C, Mariani L, Bonginelli P, Amici S, De Sio L, Fanelli M, Torino F, Bonsignori M, Gasparini G (2006) Trastuzumab in combination with gemcitabine and vinorelbine as second-line therapy for HER-2/neu overexpressing metastatic breast cancer. Oncol Rep 16(2):393–398
25. Bartsch R, Wenzel C, Altorjai G, Pluschnig U, Bachleitner-Hoffmann T, Locker GJ, Rudas M, Mader R, Zielinski CC, Steger GG (2007) Results from an observational trial with oral vinorelbine and trastuzumab in advanced breast cancer. Breast Cancer Res Treat 102 (3):375–381
26. Montemurro F, Donadio M, Clavarezza M, Redana S, Jacomuzzi ME, Valabrega G, Danese S, Vietti-Ramus G, Durando A, Venturini M, Aglietta M (2006) Outcome of patients with HER2-positive advanced breast cancer progressing during trastuzumab-based therapy. Oncologist 11(4):318–324
27. Orlando L, Cardillo A, Ghisini R, Rocca A, Balduzzi A, Torrisi R, Peruzzotti G, Goldhirsch A, Pietri E, Colleoni M (2006) Trastuzumab in combination with metronomic cyclophosphamide and methotrexate in patients with HER2 positive metastatic breast cancer. BMC Cancer 15(6):225
28. Bachelot T, Mauriac L, Delcambre C, Maillart P, Veyret C, Mouret-Reynier M, Van Praagh I, Chollet P (2007) Efficacy and safety of trastuzumab plus vinorelbine as second-line treatment for women with HER-2-positive metastatic breast cancer beyond disease progression. ASCO Annual Meeting Proceedings Part I. J Clin Oncol 25(18S):1094
29. Bartsch R, Wenzel C, Altorjai G, Pluschnig U, Rudas M, Mader RM, Gnant M, Zielinski CC, Steger GG (2007) Capecitabine and trastuzumabtrastuzumab in heavily pretreated metastatic breast cancer. J Clin Oncol 25(25):3853–3858
30. Metro G, Mottolese M, Di Cosimo S, Papaldo P, Ferretti G, Carlini P, Cianciulli AM, Giannarelli D, Cognetti F, Fabi A (2007) Activity of trastuzumab (t) beyond disease progression in HER2 over-expressing metastatic breast cancer (MBC). ASCO Annual Meeting Proceedings Part I. J Clin Oncol 25(18S):1066
31. Jackisch C, Eustermann H, Schoenegg W et al (2007) Routine clinical usage of trastuzumab (Herceptin®) in advanced breast cancer in Germany from 2001 to 2006, San Antonio Breast Cancer Symposium 2007, Abstract 2134

32. Bartsch R, Wenzel C, Hussian D et al (2006) Analysis of trastuzumab and chemotherapy in advanced breast cancer after the failure of at least one earlier combination: an observational study. BMC Cancer 6:63
33. Geyer CE, Forster J, Lindquist D, Chan S, Romieu CG, Pienkowski T et al (2006) Lapatinib plus capecitabine for HER2-positive advanced breast cancer. N Engl J Med 355(26): 2733–2743
34. Cameron D, Casey M, Press M, Lindquist D, Pienkowski T, Romieu CG et al (2008) A phase III randomized comparison of lapatinib plus capecitabine versus capecitabine alone in women with advanced breast cancer that has progressed on trastuzumab: updated efficacy and biomarker analyses. Breast Cancer Res Treat 112(3):533–543
35. von Minckwitz G, du Bois A, Schmidt M, Maass N, Cufer T, de Jongh FE et al (2009) Trastuzumab beyond progression in human epidermal growth factor receptor 2-positive advanced breast cancer: a german breast group 26/breast international group 03-05 study. J Clin Oncol 27:1999–2006
36. Schaller G, Fuchs I, Gonsch T, Weber J, Kleine-Tebbe A, Klare P et al (2007) Phase II study of capecitabine plus trastuzumab in human epidermal growth factor receptor 2 overexpressing metastatic breast cancer pretreated with anthracyclines or taxanes. J Clin Oncol 25 (22):3246–3250
37. THOR study: a study of continued Herceptin (Trastuzumab) in combination with second line chemotherapy in patients With HER2 positive metastatic breast cancer. http://www.cancer.gov/search/ViewClinicalTrials.aspx?cdrid=542712&version=HealthProfessional&protocolsearchid=3577090
38. A study of Herceptin (Trastuzumab) in combination with 2nd-line chemotherapy in patients with HER2 positive metastatic breast cancer. http://www.cancer.gov/search/ViewClinicalTrials.aspx?cdrid=539603&version=HealthProfessional&protocolsearchid=3577090
39. O'Shaughnessy J, Blackwell KL, Burstein H, Storniolo HM, Sledge G, Baselga J et al (2008) A randomized study of lapatinib alone or in combination with trastuzumab in heavily pretreated HER2+ metastatic breast cancer progressing on trastuzumab therapy. J Clin Oncol 26(Suppl): abstract 1015
40. Gelmon KA, Fumoleau P, Verma S, Wardley AM, Conte PF, Miles D, et al (2008) Results of a phase II trial of trastuzumab (H) and pertuzumab (P) in patients (pts) with HER2-positive metastatic breast cancer (MBC) who had progressed during trastuzumab therapy. J Clin Oncol 26(Suppl): abstract 1026

Pertuzumab – a HER-2 Dimerisation Inhibitor – for the Treatment of Breast and Other Cancers

Giulia Bianchi and Luca Gianni

Abstract Pertuzumab is a recombinant humanised monoclonal antibody targeting the extracellular domain of human epidermal growth factor receptor 2 (HER-2) to block HER-2 dimerisation with other HER family members. Preclinical pertuzumab data showed activity in a number of solid tumour types, and synergistic or additive activity was also observed when pertuzumab was combined with chemotherapy or with other targeted agents, including trastuzumab and erlotinib. Pertuzumab has also been studied in the clinical setting, both as monotherapy and in combination with other agents in a variety of tumour types. Following encouraging results of a Phase II trial of pertuzumab and trastuzumab in patients with HER-2-positive metastatic breast cancer, this indication has become the focus of attention for further investigation.

1 Introduction

Pertuzumab, a recombinant humanised monoclonal antibody (MAb) targeting the extracellular domain of human epidermal growth factor receptor 2 (HER-2), is currently being investigated in a range of solid tumours. The validity of HER-2 as a target in cancer therapy has primarily been demonstrated by the efficacy of the HER-2-targeted MAb trastuzumab in treating HER-2-positive metastatic breast cancer (MBC) [1–3]. In contrast to trastuzumab, which inhibits signalling via HER-2 alone, pertuzumab is a HER-2 dimerisation inhibitor, blocking ligand-activated signalling via HER-2 heterodimers. By inhibiting receptor dimerisation,

L. Gianni (✉)
Medical Oncology, Istituto dei Tumori di Milano, Via Venezian 1, 20133 Milano, Italy
e-mail: gianni@istitutotumori.mi.it

M. Sibilia et al. (eds.), *Drugs for HER-2-positive Breast Cancer*,
Milestones in Drug Therapy, DOI 10.1007/978-3-0346-0094-1_5,

pertuzumab is anticipated to have broader HER-2 blockade than trastuzumab, and may also be useful in combination with trastuzumab and other therapies acting on the HER family due to this complementary mechanism of action.

We review the rationale for the development of pertuzumab, available preclinical data showing its mechanism of action, and completed and ongoing clinical trials in solid tumours, including breast and ovarian carcinomas.

2 The HER Family and Its Role in Cancer

The HER family consists of four structurally related members: HER1 (also known as epidermal growth factor receptor), HER-2, HER3 and HER4 [4]. Each receptor molecule consists of an extracellular ligand-binding domain, a transmembrane domain and an intracellular tyrosine kinase (TK) domain [5]. A range of HER ligands has been identified, including transforming growth factor alpha, epidermal growth factor and heregulins [4]. Binding of these ligands to the HER family causes the receptors to form homodimers and heterodimers, which in turn stimulates intrinsic TK activity through phosphorylation [6, 7]. The end result is activation or modulation of many cellular processes, including cell proliferation, differentiation, migration and survival [8, 9]. Specific pathways that are known to be activated by the HER family include the phosphoinositide 3-kinase signalling pathway, which mediates cell survival, and the mitogen-activated protein kinase pathway, which regulates cellular processes, such as gene transcription and proliferation [10].

HER-2 is unique among the HER family in that it has no known natural ligand [7]. Instead, it potentiates receptor signalling through dimerisation with other members of the family [7]. HER3 is also unusual because it lacks intrinsic TK activity, relying instead on dimerisation with other HER family members to transduce signals [4]. Dimerisation of HER family members is believed to be essential for HER activity and may play an important role in driving malignant cell growth and survival in many tumour types [11, 12]. HER-2 is constitutively active and is, therefore, the preferred heterodimerisation partner of all HER family members [13, 14].

Changes in expression and activation of HERs have been documented in a range of epithelial tumour types, including breast, lung, prostate, colorectal and ovarian cancers, and they are often associated with aggressive disease and poor clinical outcomes [15–20]. HER-2 over-expression by gene amplification has been documented in 20–25% of breast cancers [21–24], and co-expression of HER1 and HER-2 is frequently observed in ovarian cancers [25].

The involvement of the HER family in tumourigenesis, and the central role played by HER-2 in potentiating signalling of other HER molecules, makes HER-2 a logical candidate for targeted anti-cancer therapies.

3 Pertuzumab

3.1 Preclinical Data

Pertuzumab is a recombinant humanised MAb that binds to the extracellular domain of HER-2 and blocks its ability to dimerise with other HER family receptors (Fig. 1) [26]. These actions contrast with those of trastuzumab – an established HER-2-targeted MAb – which binds to a different section of the HER-2 extracellular domain and does not affect the ability of HER-2 to dimerise with other members of the HER family (Fig. 1). The complementary actions of pertuzumab and trastuzumab at HER-2 suggest that they have synergistic activity.

3.1.1 Pertuzumab Alone

The pharmacokinetics of pertuzumab have been examined in mice, rats and cynomolgus monkeys [27]. Studies involving single and multiple doses of pertuzumab

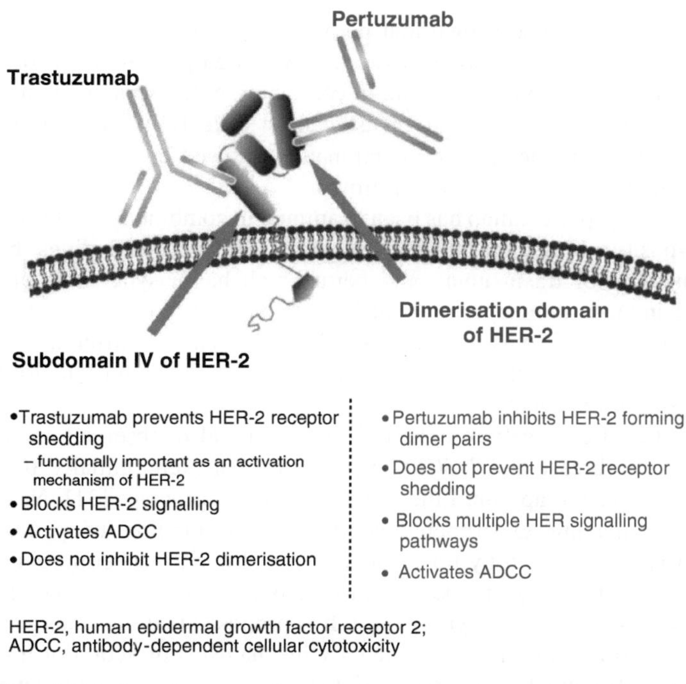

Fig. 1 Differential binding of pertuzumab and trastuzumab to the extracellular domain of HER-2, and the potential for the monoclonal antibodies to act synergistically

revealed biphasic disposition consistent with a two-compartment model. The analyses indicated that pertuzumab has a distribution phase of <1 day, a terminal half-life of ~10 days and a volume of distribution of ~40 mL/kg. The safety of the drug was evaluated in cynomolgus monkeys at doses of 15, 50 and 150 mg/kg. Treatment was well tolerated at all dose levels and the only notable adverse event (AE) was diarrhoea. The incidence of diarrhoea was generally higher in animals receiving 150 mg/kg and resolved following treatment cessation. No cardiac toxicity was noted in animal studies.

In vitro studies in cell lines derived from breast and prostate tumours show that pertuzumab inhibits the formation of HER-2-containing dimers and diminishes ligand-activated HER-2 signalling via Akt and mitogen-activated protein kinase (Erk1 and Erk2) pathways [10]. Pertuzumab has also shown activity in a variety of mouse xenograft models, including breast, lung and prostate [10, 28]. In contrast to trastuzumab, however, the activity of pertuzumab in tumour models is independent of HER-2 protein-expression level, with <80% growth inhibition observed in low HER-2-expressing breast cancer explants [10].

3.1.2 Pertuzumab in Combination with Other Targeted Agents

In vitro studies have also shown that pertuzumab augments the activity of other inhibitors of the HER pathway. Friess et al. evaluated pertuzumab and the HER1 TK inhibitor erlotinib, both alone and in combination, in explanted non-small-cell lung cancer (NSCLC) cells and breast cancer cells [29]. They observed that compared with monotherapy, the combination showed additive or greater than additive inhibitory effects on tumour growth.

More recently, pertuzumab has been examined in combination with trastuzumab in HER-2-positive breast and NSCLC xenografts [30, 31]. The findings showed that the combination of trastuzumab and pertuzumab has a synergistic anti-tumour effect and induces tumour regression in both xenograft models that cannot be achieved by either MAb as monotherapy (Fig. 2) [31]. The differential effects of trastuzumab and pertuzumab on HER-2 dimerisation may contribute to the synergistic activity of the agents.

Synergistic effects between these MAbs were also observed in mice with HER-2-positive breast and NSCLC xenografts that were initially treated with trastuzumab monotherapy until the tumour started to progress [31]. Near-infrared fluorescence imaging experiments confirmed that binding of pertuzumab to tumours was not impaired by trastuzumab pretreatment. Furthermore, the authors showed by in vitro assay that both trastuzumab and pertuzumab potently activate antibody-dependent cellular cytotoxicity. It is proposed that the synergistic effects are due to the differing but complementary mechanisms of action of trastuzumab and pertuzumab, namely prevention of formation of $p95^{HER\text{-}2}$ (a truncated and constitutively active form of HER-2 [32]) and inhibition of HER-2 dimerisation, respectively [31].

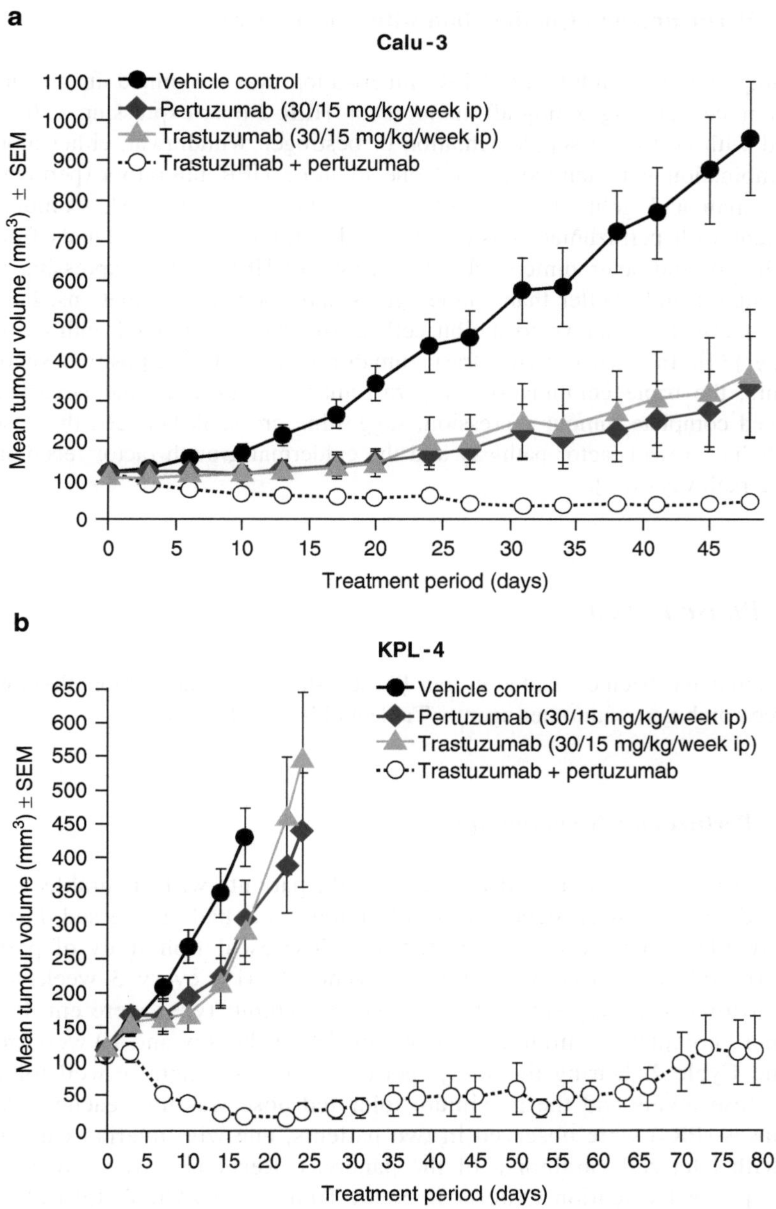

Fig. 2 Combination of trastuzumab and pertuzumab induces tumour regression in (**a**) non-small-cell lung cancer (Calu-3) and (**b**) breast (KPL-4) xenograft tumour models [31]. NB permission will be required to reproduce this figure

3.1.3 Pertuzumab in Combination with Chemotherapy

The importance of inhibiting HER dimerisation was examined in a study in which mice carrying xenograft tumours of HER-2-over-expressing cells were treated with oestrogen supplementation or oestrogen withdrawal, either alone or in combination with tamoxifen and one to three HER inhibitors (pertuzumab, trastuzumab and gefitinib, a HER1-targeted TK inhibitor) [33]. Combination treatment with pertuzumab, trastuzumab and gefitinib to block signals from all HER homo- and heterodimers inhibited growth of HER-2-over-expressing xenografts significantly better than single agents and doublet combinations. Pertuzumab has also been shown to inhibit cell growth when combined with cytotoxic therapy [34]. In mice carrying trastuzumab-resistant, HER-2-positive xenograft tumours, the triple combination of pertuzumab, trastuzumab and bevacizumab achieved complete tumour regression, suggesting crosstalk between the vascular endothelial growth factor pathway and the epidermal growth factor receptor and HER-2 pathways [35].

3.2 Phase I Data

Pertuzumab has been evaluated in four Phase I studies: in one as monotherapy and in three combined with other agents (Table 1) [36–45, 47–49].

3.2.1 Pertuzumab Monotherapy

In an initial study conducted by Agus et al., patients with incurable, locally advanced, recurrent or metastatic solid tumours that had progressed during or after standard therapy were recruited to a dose-escalation study of pertuzumab (0.5–15 mg/kg) administered intravenously (iv) every 3 weeks (q3w) [36]. A total of 21 patients with a variety of tumour types were enrolled, of whom 19 completed a minimum of two cycles of therapy and 10 were treated beyond Cycle 2. During the study, pertuzumab was generally well tolerated at all dose levels and the maximum tolerated dose was not reached. Partial responses (PRs) were observed in two patients, one with ovarian cancer and one with islet-cell carcinoma of the pancreas. Responses were documented by Response Evaluation Criteria In Solid Tumours (RECIST) [50] after 1.5 and 6 months of pertuzumab therapy, respectively, and lasted for 11 and 10 months, respectively. Stable disease (SD) lasting for >2.5 months was observed in six patients. The pharmacokinetics of pertuzumab was similar to other humanised immunoglobulin G antibodies, supporting a 3-week dosing regimen.

Table 1 Clinical trials of pertuzumab, alone and in combination with other agents

Indication	Dose/regimen	No. of patients	Key efficacy findings (for completed studies)
Phase I: monotherapy			
Advanced solid tumours	Pertuzumab 0.5, 2, 5, 10 and 15 mg/kg	21	PRs observed in 2 patients: 1 patient with ovarian cancer experienced a PR of 10 months after 6 months' therapy and 1 patient with pancreatic islet-cell carcinoma experienced a PR of 11 months following 1.5 months' therapy; 6 patients experienced SD of >2.5 months (range 2.6–5.5) [36]
Phase I: combination therapy			
Advanced solid tumours	Pertuzumab 1,050 mg + capecitabine 825, 1,000, 1,250 mg/m^2	18	Of 18 patients evaluated for response, 11 achieved SD [37]
	Pertuzumab 1,050 mg + docetaxel 60, 75 mg/m^2 Pertuzumab 420 mg[a] + docetaxel 75, 100 mg/m^2	19	SD was observed at 4 cycles in >50% of patients treated. Confirmed radiological PR with >50% decline in PSA in a patient with HRPC was observed [38]
Advanced NSCLC	Pertuzumab 420 mg[a] + erlotinib 100, 150 mg/day	9	Study closed, final results expected 2009 [39]
Phase II: monotherapy			
Advanced ovarian cancer	Cohort 1: pertuzumab 420 mg[a]	61	Of 117 patients assessable for efficacy, 5 (4.3%) had a PR, 8 (6.8%) had SD for ≥6 months and 10 had CA125 reduction of ≥50%. Median PFS was 6.6 weeks [40]
	Cohort 2: pertuzumab 1,050 mg	62	
MBC with low HER-2 expression	Arm A: pertuzumab 420 mg[a]	41	10% of patients had either a PR or SD for ≥6 months [41]
	Arm B: pertuzumab 1,050 mg	37	
HRPC, chemotherapy naïve	Cohort 1: pertuzumab 420 mg[a]	35	Pertuzumab has no clinically significant single-agent activity in castrate patients with HRPC at either dose level [42]
	Cohort 2: pertuzumab 1,050 mg	33	
HRPC pre-treated with docetaxel	Pertuzumab 420 mg[a]	41	Of 30 efficacy-assessable patients, 5 had SD for ≥23 weeks; 1/5 had SD for 36 weeks. No patients had CR or PR [43]
Advanced, recurrent NSCLC	Pertuzumab 420 mg[a]	43	None of the 43 patients experienced a response [44]

(continued)

Table 1 (continued)

Indication	Dose/regimen	No. of patients	Key efficacy findings (for completed studies)
Phase II: combination therapy			
HER-2-positive MBC	Pertuzumab 420 mg[a] + trastuzumab 2 mg/kg qw, 6 mg/kg q3w	66	CBR was 50%, ORR was 24.2%; 5 patients (7.6%) experienced a CR, 11 (16.7%) experienced a PR and 17 (25.8%) experienced SD for ≥6 months. Median PFS was 5.5 months [45, 46]
HER-2-positive MBC	Pertuzumab 420 mg[a] + trastuzumab (LD 6/8 mg/m^2), 6 mg/m^2	11	ORR was 18%. 2 patients had a PR, 3 had SD, 6 had PD. Median TTP was 6 weeks [47]
Platinum-resistant ovarian, peritoneal or fallopian tube cancer	Gemcitabine 800 mg/m^2 ± pertuzumab/placebo 420 mg[a]	65 65	Median PFS not significantly different between gemcitabine + placebo vs gemcitabine + pertuzumab arms (2.6 vs 3.0 months, respectively); PFS at 4 months was 34% vs 49% [48]. Retrospective analysis by HER3 mRNA level showed an efficacy signal
Platinum-sensitive ovarian cancer	Carboplatin-based chemotherapy[b] ± pertuzumab 420 mg[a]	150	Median PFS not significantly different between chemotherapy alone or with pertuzumab. Slight trend towards improved PFS was seen in patients with lower HER3 mRNA levels [49]

[a]LD of 840 mg
[b]Maintenance dose q3w
CBR clinical benefit rate, *CR* complete response, *HER* human epidermal growth factor receptor, *HRPC* hormone-refractory prostate cancer, *LD* loading dose, *MBC* metastatic breast cancer, *NSCLC* non-small-cell lung cancer, *ORR* objective response rate, *PD* progressive disease, *PFS* progression-free survival, *PR* partial response, *PSA* prostate-specific antigen, *qw* weekly, *q3w* 3-weekly, *SD* stable disease, *TTP* time to progression

3.2.2 Pertuzumab Combination Therapy

A study of pertuzumab in combination with docetaxel – an anti-mitotic chemotherapy – was conducted to determine the maximum tolerated dose, dose-limiting toxicities and any pharmacokinetic interactions between the two compounds [38]. From the study, the recommended dose for this combination was established as docetaxel 75 mg/m^2 and pertuzumab 420 mg following a loading dose of 840 mg.

SD was observed after four cycles in more than half of the patients treated; confirmed radiological PR with a >50% decline in prostate-specific antigen was observed in a patient with hormone-refractory prostate cancer.

Pertuzumab has also been examined in combination with capecitabine – an oral fluoropyrimidine that is metabolised to 5-fluorouracil – in patients with advanced malignancies [37]. Patients were treated in three sequential cohorts with pertuzumab at a fixed dose of 1,050 mg given iv on day 1 plus escalating-dose oral capecitabine (825, 1,000, 1,250 mg/m^2) twice daily on days 1–14 of each 21-day treatment cycle. The combination of capecitabine and pertuzumab was well tolerated at all dose levels and no dose-limiting toxicities were observed. There was no apparent change in the pharmacokinetics of capecitabine or pertuzumab when administered together. Clinical activity was observed, with SD reported in 11 of 18 patients.

Initial findings from a Phase I combination trial of pertuzumab 420 mg q3w (840 mg loading dose) with oral erlotinib 100 mg in patients with NSCLC indicate that this combination is also well tolerated, with the most frequent AEs being rash and diarrhoea [39]. These AEs were mostly mild, with grade 3 rash and diarrhoea experienced by 27% and 7% of patients, respectively. A second phase of the trial, in which patients will receive pertuzumab in combination with erlotinib 150 mg, is now underway.

3.2.3 Pertuzumab Dosing and Scheduling

The Phase I trials established effective and tolerable dosing schedules for pertuzumab that were used in further trials. The optimum dosing schedules were either a loading dose of 840 mg followed by 420 mg q3w or a higher dose of 1,050 mg q3w, which has been used in some Phase II studies in breast cancer and ovarian cancer [40, 41].

3.3 Clinical Trials in Breast Cancer

Following the signals of clinical activity with pertuzumab that were observed in the Phase I clinical trials in advanced solid tumours, Phase II trials were initiated in more specific tumour types, namely cancers of the breast, ovary, prostate and lung. One of the first trials involved 79 patients with MBC with low HER-2 expression [41, 51]. Patients were randomised to receive iv pertuzumab q3w, either at 420 mg with a loading dose of 840 mg ($n = 41$) or at 1,050 mg ($n = 37$). The results of this study showed only limited efficacy in HER-2-normal patients: only two patients, both receiving the lower dose of pertuzumab, showed a PR; SD was observed in 44% of patients who received pertuzumab 420 mg and in 38% of those who received the 1,050 mg dose.

Based on excellent preclinical results in combination with trastuzumab in HER-2-positive tumour models and the limited efficacy seen in HER-2-normal patients, the focus of investigations moved to HER-2-positive breast cancer. In an initial small study, 11 patients with measurable HER-2-positive MBC who had received up to three trastuzumab-based regimens received trastuzumab 8 or 6 mg/kg and pertuzumab 840 mg iv loading dose in Cycle 1 followed by trastuzumab 6 mg/kg and pertuzumab 420 mg q3w in subsequent cycles [47]. In total, patients received 64 cycles of trastuzumab plus pertuzumab. The objective response rate (ORR) was 18%: two patients had a PR, three had SD and six had progressive disease. The median time to progression was 6 weeks. Overall, the combination of trastuzumab and pertuzumab was well tolerated, with grade 1 and grade 2 diarrhoea (according to the National Cancer Institute Common Terminology Criteria for Adverse Events) being the most common AE, occurring in 18% and 27% of patients, respectively. Unexpectedly, echocardiogram and cardiac magnetic resonance analysis revealed left ventricular systolic dysfunction in six patients (54%; three grade 1, two grade 2 and one grade 3). The majority of cardiac toxicity observed in the study was asymptomatic and reversible; however, as the long-term effects of these cardiac effects are not known, further investigation is warranted to define overall risks and benefits. A larger second study, also investigating the combination of trastuzumab and pertuzumab in trastuzumab-pre-treated patients, did not confirm these findings [45, 46]. In this study, 66 patients with HER-2-positive MBC that had progressed during prior trastuzumab therapy received weekly trastuzumab (4 mg/kg loading dose then 2 mg/kg weekly) or 8 mg/kg loading dose then 6 mg/kg q3w, and pertuzumab q3w (840 mg loading dose then 420 mg q3w). The results from this trial were encouraging: the clinical benefit rate was 50% and the ORR was 24.2% (Table 2) [45]. Five patients (7.6%) experienced a complete response, 11 patients (16.7%) experienced a PR and 17 patients (25.8%) experienced SD for ≥6 months. The median progression-free survival (PFS) was 5.5 months. Due to these promising results, a third cohort of patients has been recruited, using similar inclusion and exclusion criteria, to assess the activity of pertuzumab monotherapy in this population. Following documented progression during pertuzumab monotherapy, trastuzumab could be added to continuing pertuzumab treatment. To date, 29 patients have been recruited, with a clinical benefit rate of 11.1% (including 7.4% PR and 3.7% SD of ≥8 cycles) [52]. Fifteen of these 29 patients have had trastuzumab added to their continuing pertuzumab

Table 2 Response rates in patients ($n = 66$) with human epidermal growth factor 2-receptor positive metastatic breast cancer [45]

Best overall response	*n* (%)
Responders	33 (50)
Non-responders	33 (50)
Complete response	5 (7.6)
Partial response	11 (16.7)
Stable disease ≥8 cycles	17 (25.8)
Progressive disease	33 (50)

following documented progression, with a 20% PR rate. It is particularly noteworthy that these patients who had progressed during two prior lines of anti-HER-2 therapy responded to treatment with a combination of pertuzumab and trastuzumab. However, at the time of this analysis, two patients receiving pertuzumab monotherapy and four patients receiving pertuzumab and trastuzumab had not yet reached eight cycles of assessment to reach the overall best response end point. Further data are eagerly awaited.

Overall, the combination of trastuzumab and pertuzumab was well tolerated and AEs were mild to moderate. The most frequent AEs (grade 1/2 [grade 3/4]) in the original two cohorts treated with pertuzumab and trastuzumab were diarrhoea (64% [3%]), fatigue (33% [0%]), nausea (27% [0%]), skin rash (26% [2%]) and headache (20% [0%]), which were similar to those experienced by patients in the third cohort receiving this combination (diarrhoea 27% [7%], nausea 27% [0%], vomiting 27% [0%] and fatigue 27% [7%]). In patients who received pertuzumab monotherapy, the most frequent AEs were also diarrhoea (48% [3%]), nausea (34% [0%]), vomiting (24% [0%]) and fatigue (17% [3%]). These AEs are most likely caused by a reduction in HER1:HER-2 dimers and are much less severe than the gastrointestinal and skin toxicities associated with other agents that block HER1 signalling, such as lapatinib and cetuximab [53, 54]. In contrast to the trial conducted by Portera et al. [47], only three patients had a decrease in left ventricular ejection fraction (LVEF) of $\geq$10% points and <50% absolute value, and none of these patents experienced any clinical symptoms related to the cardiac changes. In the third cohort, two patients receiving pertuzumab monotherapy and one patient receiving the combination experienced asymptomatic LVEF falls, none of which required treatment [52]. Differences between the studies conducted by Portera et al. [47] and Baselga et al. [45, 46, 52], including the exclusion criteria and criteria to evaluate the decline in LVEF, may explain the different outcomes. In particular, it should be noted that patients who had experienced a decrease in LVEF during trastuzumab therapy or had a history of hypertension were eligible for the Portera trial [47] but were excluded from the study conducted by Baselga et al. [45, 46].

The efficacy of pertuzumab in HER-2-positive breast cancer is now being tested in a Phase III study – CLEOPATRA (CLinical Evaluation Of Pertuzumab And TRAstuzumab). This study has been designed to investigate PFS in 800 previously untreated women with HER-2-positive MBC receiving trastuzumab (8 mg/kg loading dose then 6 mg/kg q3w) plus docetaxel (75 mg/m^2 q3w $\times$ 6) with or without pertuzumab (840 mg loading dose then 420 mg q3w). A Phase II study of neo-adjuvant treatment with pertuzumab plus trastuzumab (with or without docetaxel) in HER-2-positive early breast cancer (NEOSPHERE) completed accrual in the summer of 2009. Two further studies are currently in development: a randomised Phase II trial of trastuzumab and capecitabine with or without pertuzumab in patients with HER-2-positive MBC who had progressed after one line of trastuzumab-based therapy in the metastatic setting (PHEREXA), and a randomised Phase II trial to evaluate pertuzumab and trastuzumab given with either anthracycline- or non-anthracycline-based chemotherapy as neo-adjuvant therapy for HER-2-positive breast cancer.

3.4 Clinical Trials in Ovarian Cancer

The efficacy of pertuzumab has also been evaluated in ovarian cancer. In an initial trial, the efficacy of pertuzumab as monotherapy was examined in patients with advanced, refractory ovarian cancer who had been heavily pre-treated [40]. Patients received either a loading dose of pertuzumab 840 mg iv followed by 420 mg q3w ($n = 61$) or 1,050 mg q3w ($n = 62$). The primary end point of the study was response rate. Tumour biopsies were obtained in the low-dose group to perform an exploratory analysis of phosphorylated HER-2 (pHER2). Efficacy was assessed in 122 patients. The ORR was 4.3%, with an additional 41% achieving SD. The median PFS was 6.6 weeks and median overall survival was 52.7 weeks.

The biopsy findings suggested an association between the presence of pHER2 and efficacy. Analysis of 28 samples in which HER-2 status could be determined revealed eight (29%) with evidence of phosphorylation. Overall, more patients with pHER2 had SD compared with those without phosphorylation (75% vs 25%, respectively) and more patients without pHER2 experienced progression (65% vs 12.5%). Furthermore, the median time to progression was longer in the pHER2 cohort compared with the cohort without pHER2 (20.9 vs 5.8 weeks, respectively). Pertuzumab was well tolerated in the study. Diarrhoea was reported in 69.1% of patients and five patients had asymptomatic LVEF decreases of <50%.

The findings from this preliminary trial prompted further investigation into the efficacy of pertuzumab in patients with ovarian cancer. Makhija et al. presented findings from a trial investigating the efficacy of pertuzumab in platinum-resistant epithelial ovarian cancer [48]. Patients who had previously received up to one therapeutic intervention were randomised to gemcitabine 800 mg/m^2 on days 1 and 8 of a 28-day cycle, with either pertuzumab (840 mg initial dose followed by 420 mg iv q3w) or placebo. The primary outcome was PFS, with tumour response assessed using RECIST. In addition, HER-2 activation-related expression profiles were examined.

A total of 130 patients received treatment. The median PFS was not significantly different between the gemcitabine plus placebo arm compared with the gemcitabine plus pertuzumab arm (2.6 vs 3.0 months, respectively; $p = 0.07$); the 4-month PFS rate was 34% versus 49%, respectively. The combination was generally well tolerated. The most frequent AEs in the pertuzumab patients were fatigue, nausea, diarrhoea, back pain, grade 3/4 neutropenia, skin rash, headache, stomatitis, epistaxis and rhinorrhoea. Clinically significant congestive heart failure was reported in one patient who received pertuzumab but there was no imbalance in LVEF results between the treatment arms. The exploratory analysis of HER-2 activation-related expression profiles indicated that low HER3 mRNA levels may be a predictive marker in this patient population [55, 56]. Women who had low HER3 mRNA levels ($n = 61$) had longer PFS if they received gemcitabine plus pertuzumab rather than gemcitabine plus placebo (5.3 vs 1.4 months, respectively; hazard ratio 0.34). Conversely, those with high HER3 mRNA levels ($n = 61$) had shorter PFS if they received gemcitabine plus pertuzumab rather than gemcitabine plus placebo (2.8 vs 5.5 months, respectively; hazard ratio 1.48). A similar relationship was noted for HER3 mRNA levels and overall survival.

A trial of pertuzumab in combination with either carboplatin/paclitaxel or carboplatin/gemcitabine in patients with relapsed platinum-sensitive ovarian cancer has been performed. The data indicate that pertuzumab in combination with carboplatin-based chemotherapy is well tolerated, with no new safety signals or clinically significant cardiac toxicity [49]. Pertuzumab does not appear to enhance the activity of chemotherapy in this patient group; however, retrospective analyses in those patients with sensitive ovarian cancer who had a relatively a short treatment-free interval (6–12 months) show that low HER3 mRNA expression may be associated with benefit from chemotherapy plus pertuzumab, similar to the reported findings of Amler et al. [55, 56] in patients with resistant ovarian cancer. This may be due to negative feedback loop in which HER-2/HER3 dimerisation leads to downregulation of, and therefore lower expression of, HER3 [56].

3.5 Clinical Trials in Other Malignancies

Clinical trials of pertuzumab have been conducted in other tumours, including prostate cancer and NSCLC, but the results have been mixed. A study conducted by Agus et al. in 41 patients with hormone-refractory prostate cancer failed to show evidence of response [43]. Among the 30 patients in whom efficacy was assessed, 17% achieved SD, remaining progression free for $\geq$23 weeks. Retrospective analysis suggested that survival was prolonged with pertuzumab treatment compared with historic controls with similar baseline prognostic features. A separate study in castrate patients with hormone-refractory prostate cancer treated with pertuzumab 420 mg (840 mg loading dose) or 1,050 mg iv q3w failed to show any clinical response, as defined by a 50% decline in prostate-specific antigen [42].

A trial of pertuzumab in NSCLC revealed no responses among 43 patients. Eighteen (41.9%) and nine patients (20.9%) had SD at 6 and 12 weeks, respectively, and the median PFS was 6 weeks [44]. The authors concluded that further clinical development of pertuzumab should focus on rational combinations of pertuzumab with other drugs active in NSCLC. One such approach would be a combination of therapies that inhibit different aspects of the HER family. Pertuzumab has been investigated in combination with the HER1 TK inhibitor erlotinib in a Phase I dose-escalation study in patients with previously treated NSCLC [39]. No dose-limiting toxicities were observed in either the first cohort receiving an 840 mg loading dose of pertuzumab followed by 420 mg three times a week thereafter and erlotinib 100 mg once daily, or the second cohort receiving erlotinib 150 mg once daily combined with the same dose of pertuzumab, which was, therefore, selected as the optimum dose level for the combination [39]. At the time of analysis, the six patients in Cohort 1 had best tumour responses of two with PRs, two with SD and two with disease progression, while the seven evaluable patients in Cohort 2 achieved responses of one with PR, three with SD and three with disease progression. Two further patients in Cohort 2 had not yet reached the best tumour response end point. A Phase II study of pertuzumab in combination with erlotinib is currently ongoing (NCT00855894; http://www.clinicaltrial.gov/ct2/show/NCT00855894?term=pertuzumab&cond=cancer&rank=8) in patients with relapsed or previously treated NSCLC.

4 Conclusions and Future Directions

Pertuzumab represents a novel approach to the treatment of cancers in which HER pathways are disrupted. As a HER-2 dimerisation inhibitor, the activities of pertuzumab would be anticipated to extend beyond its role as a HER-2-targeted agent. By blocking receptor dimerisation, pertuzumab is anticipated to have broader applicability than therapies acting on individual HERs and could also act synergistically when used in combination with such agents.

Preclinical data indicated that pertuzumab inhibits growth in a wide range of tumour models, with evidence that growth inhibition was independent of HER-2 levels. Phase I/II monotherapy trials suggested that, despite the preclinical data in HER-2-negative tumour types, investigations should focus on HER-2-positive tumours as well as combinations of pertuzumab with other agents targeting the HER system in both HER-2-positive and HER-2-normal tumours.

Investigations of pertuzumab in lung and prostate cancers indicated a lack of single-agent activity, suggesting that pertuzumab monotherapy in these tumour types would not be sensible. The potential for pertuzumab to provide benefits when used in combination with other agents, particularly those acting on different members of the HER family, remains a possibility. While trials of pertuzumab in combination with other HER family inhibitors in NSCLC are ongoing, it seems no further investigations into the efficacy of pertuzumab in prostate cancers will proceed.

The applicability of pertuzumab in the treatment of ovarian cancer is also unclear. Response rates from a trial combining pertuzumab with gemcitabine were disappointing, although subgroup analyses from this trial suggested a specific subpopulation with low levels of HER3 mRNA may benefit from therapy. Further investigation of responsive subpopulations in different tumour types is warranted.

Based on the encouraging Phase II findings for pertuzumab in HER-2-positive breast cancer, this indication has become the focus of attention for further investigation with more trials now underway. Pertuzumab is currently being evaluated in a large, first-line, randomised, Phase III trial of women with metastatic HER-2-positive MBC. In this trial, women will be randomised to receive docetaxel and trastuzumab with either placebo or pertuzumab. A Phase II study of neo-adjuvant treatment with pertuzumab plus trastuzumab (with or without docetaxel) in HER-2-positive early breast cancer has just completed accrual and will be ready for analysis by the summer of 2010. A Phase II trial (PHEREXA) is in preparation to investigate the addition of pertuzumab to trastuzumab and capecitabine treatment in second-line trastuzumab-pre-treated patients. Another Phase II trial, to assess the combination of pertuzumab and trastuzumab given with chemotherapy in the neo-adjuvant setting to treat patients with HER-2-positive breast cancer, is also in development. It is anticipated that, together, these trials will determine whether the synergy noted in early development translates into clinical benefits in these patient populations, and clarify whether pertuzumab in combination with trastuzumab and chemotherapy warrants investigation in the post-surgical setting.

Acknowledgements The authors thank Lucy Kanan and Eleanor Steele for medical writing assistance in revising the first-draft manuscript and collation of review comments, funded by F. Hoffmann-La Roche Ltd.

References

1. Smith IE (2001) Efficacy and safety of Herceptin in women with metastatic breast cancer: results from pivotal clinical studies. Anticancer Drugs 12(Suppl 4):S3–S10
2. Slamon DJ, Leyland-Jones B, Shak S, Fuchs H, Paton V, Bajamonde A, Fleming T, Eiermann W, Wolter J, Pegram M et al (2001) Use of chemotherapy plus a monoclonal antibody against HER2 for metastatic breast cancer that overexpresses HER2. N Engl J Med 344:783–792
3. Marty M, Cognetti F, Maraninchi D, Snyder R, Mauriac L, Tubiana-Hulin M, Chan S, Grimes D, Antón A, Lluch A et al (2005) Randomized phase II trial of the efficacy and safety of trastuzumab combined with docetaxel in patients with human epidermal growth factor receptor 2-positive metastatic breast cancer administered as first-line treatment: the M77001 study group. J Clin Oncol 23:4265–4274
4. Yarden Y, Sliwkowski MX (2001) Untangling the ErbB signalling network. Nat Rev Mol Cell Biol 2:127–137
5. Grünwald V, Hidalgo M (2002) The epidermal growth factor receptor: a new target for anticancer therapy. Curr Probl Cancer 26:109–164
6. Pinkas-Kramarski R, Soussan L, Waterman H, Levkowitz G, Alroy I, Klapper L, Lavi S, Seger R, Ratzkin BJ, Sela M et al (1996) Diversification of Neu differentiation factor and epidermal growth factor signaling by combinatorial receptor interactions. EMBO J 15: 2452–2467
7. Tzahar E, Yarden Y (1998) The ErbB-2/HER2 oncogenic receptor of adenocarcinomas: from orphanhood to multiple stromal ligands. Biochim Biophys Acta 1377:M25–M37
8. Cho HS, Mason K, Ramyar KX, Stanley AM, Gabelli SB, Denney DW Jr, Leahy DJ (2003) Structure of the extracellular region of HER2 alone and in complex with the Herceptin Fab. Nature 421:756–760
9. Zhao YY, Sawyer DR, Baliga RR, Opel DJ, Han X, Marchionni MA, Kelly RA (1998) Neuregulins promote survival and growth of cardiac myocytes. Persistence of ErbB2 and ErbB4 expression in neonatal and adult ventricular myocytes. J Biol Chem 273:10261–10269
10. Agus DB, Akita RW, Fox WD, Lewis GD, Higgins B, Pisacane PI, Lofgren JA, Tindell C, Evans DP, Maiese K et al (2002) Targeting ligand-activated ErbB2 signaling inhibits breast and prostate tumor growth. Cancer Cell 2:127–137
11. Sundaresan S, Roberts PE, King KL, Sliwkowski MX, Mather JP (1998) Biological response to ErbB ligands in nontransformed cell lines correlates with a specific pattern of receptor expression. Endocrinology 139:4756–4764
12. Tzahar E, Waterman H, Chen X, Levkowitz G, Karunagaran D, Lavi S, Ratzkin BJ, Yarden Y (1996) A hierarchical network of interreceptor interactions determines signal transduction by

Neu differentiation factor/neuregulin and epidermal growth factor. Mol Cell Biol 16: 5276–5287

13. Burgess AW, Cho H-S, Eigenbrot C, Ferguson KM, Garrett TPJ, Leahy DJ, Lemmon MA, Sliwkowski MX, Ward CW, Yokoyama S (2003) An open-and-shut case? Recent insights into the activation of EGF/ErbB receptors. Mol Cell 12:541–552
14. Graus-Porta D, Beerli RR, Daly JM, Hynes NE (1997) ErbB-2, the preferred heterodimerization partner of all ErbB receptors, is a mediator of lateral signaling. EMBO J 16:1647–1655
15. Campiglio M, Ali S, Knyazev PG, Ullrich A (1999) Characteristics of EGFR family-mediated HRG signals in human ovarian cancer. J Cell Biochem 73:522–532
16. Holbro T, Beerli RR, Maurer F, Koziczak M, Barbas CF III, Hynes NE (2003) The ErbB2/ErbB3 heterodimer functions as an oncogenic unit: ErbB2 requires ErbB3 to drive breast tumor cell proliferation. Proc Natl Acad Sci USA 100:8933–8938
17. Kim HG, Kassis J, Souto JC, Turner T, Wells A (1999) EGF receptor signaling in prostate morphogenesis and tumorigenesis. Histol Histopathol 14:1175–1182
18. Maurer CA, Friess H, Kretschmann B, Zimmermann A, Stauffer A, Baer HU, Korc M, Büchler MW (1998) Increased expression of erbB3 in colorectal cancer is associated with concomitant increase in the level of erbB2. Hum Pathol 29:771–777
19. Meert A-P, Martin B, Delmotte P, Berghmans T, Lafitte J-J, Mascaux C, Paesmans M, Steels E, Verdebout J-M, Sculier J-P (2002) The role of EGF-R expression on patient survival in lung cancer: a systematic review with meta-analysis. Eur Respir J 20:975–981
20. Witton CJ, Reeves JR, Going JJ, Cooke TG, Bartlett JM (2003) Expression of the HER1-4 family of receptor tyrosine kinases in breast cancer. J Pathol 200:290–297
21. Owens MA, Horten BC, Da Silva MM (2004) HER2 amplification ratios by fluorescence in situ hybridization and correlation with immunohistochemistry in a cohort of 6556 breast cancer tissues. Clin Breast Cancer 5:63–69
22. Ross JS, Fletcher JA, Bloom KJ, Linette GP, Stec J, Symmans WF, Pusztai L, Hortobagyi GN (2004) Targeted therapy in breast cancer. The HER-2/neu gene and protein. Mol Cell Proteomics 3:379–398
23. Wolff AC, Hammond MEH, Schwartz JN, Hagerty KL, Allred DC, Cote RJ, Dowsett M, Fitzgibbons PL, Hanna WM, Langer A et al (2007) American Society of Clinical Oncology/College of American Pathologists guideline recommendations for human epidermal growth factor receptor 2 testing in breast cancer. J Clin Oncol 25:118–145
24. Yaziji H, Goldstein LC, Barry TS, Werling R, Hwang H, Ellis GK, Gralow JR, Livingston RB, Gown AM (2004) HER-2 testing in breast cancer using parallel tissue-based methods. JAMA 291:1972–1977
25. Bast RC Jr, Pusztai L, Kerns BJ, MacDonald JA, Jordan P, Daly L, Boyer CM, Mendelsohn J, Berchuck A (1998) Coexpression of the HER-2 gene product, p185HER-2, and epidermal growth factor receptor, p170EGF-R, on epithelial ovarian cancers and normal tissues. Hybridoma 17:313–321
26. Franklin MC, Carey KD, Vajdos FF, Leahy DJ, de Vos AM, Sliwkowski MX (2004) Insights into ErbB signaling from the structure of the ErbB2-pertuzumab complex. Cancer Cell 5: 317–328
27. Adams CW, Allison DE, Flagella K, Presta L, Clarke J, Dybdal N, McKeever K, Sliwkowski MX (2006) Humanization of a recombinant monoclonal antibody to produce a therapeutic HER dimerization inhibitor, pertuzumab. Cancer Immunol Immunother 55:717–727
28. Mendoza N, Phillips GL, Silva J, Schwall R, Wickramasinghe D (2002) Inhibition of ligand-mediated HER2 activation in androgen-independent prostate cancer. Cancer Res 62: 5485–5488
29. Friess T, Scheuer W, Hasmann M (2005) Combination treatment with erlotinib and pertuzumab against human tumor xenografts is superior to monotherapy. Clin Cancer Res 11: 5300–5309
30. Friess T, Thier M, Scheuer W, Hasmann M (2005) Combination treatment with pertuzumab and trastuzumab against Calu-3 human NSCLC xenograft tumors is superior to monotherapy.

Poster A51 presented at the 17th AACR-NCI-EORTC, Philadelphia, PA, USA, 14–18 Nov 2005

31. Friess T, Scheuer W, Hasmann M (2006) Superior antitumour activity after combination treatment with pertuzumab and trastuzumab against NSCLC and breast cancer xenograft tumours. Poster 96PD presented at the 31st ESMO Meeting, Istanbul, Turkey, 29 Sept–3 Oct 2006
32. Molina MA, Codony-Servat J, Albanell J, Rojo F, Arribas J, Baselga J (2001) Trastuzumab (Herceptin), a humanized anti-HER2 receptor monoclonal antibody, inhibits basal and activated HER2 ectodomain cleavage in breast cancer cells. Cancer Res 61:4744–4749
33. Arpino G, Gutierrez C, Weiss H, Rimawi M, Massarweh S, Bharwani L, De Placido S, Osborne CK, Schiff R (2007) Treatment of human epidermal growth factor receptor 2-overexpressing breast cancer xenografts with multiagent HER-targeted therapy. J Natl Cancer Inst 99:694–705
34. Hasmann M, Juchem R, Scheuer W, Friess T (2003) Pertuzumab (Omnitarg) potentiates antitumor effects on NSCLC xenografts without increasing toxicity when combined with cytotoxic chemotherapeutic agents. Poster B213 presented at the 15th EORTC-NCI-AACR, Boston, MA, USA, 17–21 Nov 2003
35. Alami N, Sun Y, De P, Benmassaoud AM, Wang Y, Leyland-Jones B (2009) Combination effects of herceptin, pertuzumab and bevacizumab in a HER2-overexpressing breast cancer xenograft model. Cancer Res 69(Suppl):274s
36. Agus D, Sweeney C, Morris M, Mendelson D, McNeel D, Ahmann F, Wang J, Derynck M, Kattan M, Ng K et al (2005) Efficacy and safety of single agent pertuzumab (rhuMAb 2C4), a HER dimerization inhibitor, in hormone refractory prostate cancer after failure of taxane-based therapy. Poster 4624 presented at the 41st ASCO Annual Meeting, Orlando, FL, USA, 13–17 May 2005
37. Albanell J, Montagut C, Jones ET, Pronk L, Mellado B, Beech J, Gascon P, Zugmaier G, Brewster M, Saunders MP et al (2008) A phase I study of the safety and pharmacokinetics of the combination of pertuzumab (rhuMab 2C4) and capecitabine in patients with advanced solid tumors. Clin Cancer Res 14:2726–2731
38. Attard G, Kitzen J, Blagden SP, Fong PC, Pronk LC, Zhi J, Zugmaier G, Verweij J, de Bono JS, de Jonge M (2007) A phase Ib study of pertuzumab, a recombinant humanised antibody to HER2, and docetaxel in patients with advanced solid tumours. Br J Cancer 97:1338–1343
39. Felip E, Ranson M, Cedres S, Dean E, De Droogh E, Brewster M, McNally VA, Ross G, Galdermans D (2008) A phase I, dose escalation study to determine the maximum tolerated dose of erlotinib when combined with pertuzumab in previously treated non-small-cell lung cancer patients. J Clin Oncol (Meeting Abstracts) 26:717s, abstract 19134
40. Gordon MS, Matei D, Aghajanian C, Matulonis UA, Brewer M, Fleming GF, Hainsworth JD, Garcia AA, Pegram MD, Schilder RJ et al (2006) Clinical activity of pertuzumab (rhuMAb 2C4), a HER dimerization inhibitor, in advanced ovarian cancer: potential predictive relationship with tumor HER2 activation status. J Clin Oncol 24:4324–4332
41. Cortes J, Baselga J, Wardley A, Kellokumpu-Lehtinen P, Bianchi G, Cameron D, Miles D, Salvagni S, Goeminne J-C, Gianni L (2005) Open-label, randomized, phase II study of pertuzumab (Omnitarg™) in patients with metastatic breast cancer (MBC) with low expression of HER2. Poster 3068 presented at the 41st ASCO Annual Meeting, Orlando, FL, USA, 13–17 May 2005
42. de Bono JS, Bellmunt J, Attard G, Droz JP, Miller K, Flechon A, Sternberg C, Parker C, Zugmaier G, Hersberger-Gimenez V et al (2007) Open-label phase II study evaluating the efficacy and safety of two doses of pertuzumab in castrate chemotherapy-naive patients with hormone-refractory prostate cancer. J Clin Oncol 25:257–262
43. Agus DB, Sweeney CJ, Morris MJ, Mendelson DS, McNeel DG, Ahmann FR, Wang J, Derynck MK, Ng K, Lyons B et al (2007) Efficacy and safety of single-agent pertuzumab (rhuMAb 2C4), a human epidermal growth factor receptor dimerization inhibitor, in castration-resistant prostate cancer after progression from taxane-based therapy. J Clin Oncol 25:675–681

44. Herbst RS, Davies AM, Natale RB, Dang TP, Schiller JH, Garland LL, Miller VA, Mendelson D, Van den Abbeele AD, Melenevsky Y et al (2007) Efficacy and safety of single-agent pertuzumab, a human epidermal receptor dimerization inhibitor, in patients with non small cell lung cancer. Clin Cancer Res 13:6175–6181
45. Gelmon K, Fumoleau P, Verma S, Wardley A, Conte PF, Miles D, Gianni L, McNally VA, Ross GA, Baselga J (2008) Results of a Phase II trial of trastuzumab (H) and pertuzumab (P) in patients (pts) with HER2-positive metastatic breast cancer (MBC) who had progressed during trastuzumab therapy. Poster 1026 presented at the 44th ASCO Annual Meeting, Chicago, IL, USA, 30 May–3 June 2008
46. Baselga J, Gelmon K, Verma S, Wardley A, Conte P, Miles D, Bianchi G, Cortes J, McNally VA, Ross G et al (2010) Phase II trial of pertuzumab and trastuzumab in patients with HER2-positive metastatic breast cancer that had progressed during prior trastuzumab therapy. J Clin Oncol 28(7):1138–1144
47. Portera CC, Walshe JM, Rosing DR, Denduluri N, Berman AW, Vatas U, Velarde M, Chow CK, Steinberg SM, Nguyen D et al (2008) Cardiac toxicity and efficacy of trastuzumab combined with pertuzumab in patients with trastuzumab-insensitive human epidermal growth factor receptor 2-positive metastatic breast cancer. Clin Cancer Res 14:2710–2716
48. Makhija S, Glenn D, Ueland F, Gold M, Dizon D, Paton V, Birkner M, Lin C, Derynck M, Matulonis U (2007) Results from a phase II randomized, placebo-controlled, double-blind trial suggest improved PFS with the addition of pertuzumab to gemcitabine in patients with platinum-resistant ovarian, fallopian tube, or primary peritoneal cancer. J Clin Oncol (Meeting Abstracts) 25:275s, abstract 5507
49. Kaye S, Poole CJ, Bidzinski M, Gianni L, Gorbunova V, Novikova E, Strauss A, Moczko M, McNally VA, Ross G et al (2008) A randomised Phase II study evaluating the combination of carboplatin-based chemotherapy with pertuzumab (P) versus carboplatin-based therapy alone in patients with relapsed, platinum sensitive ovarian cancer. Poster 10 presented at the 44th ASCO Annual Meeting, Chicago, IL, USA, 30 May–3 June 2008
50. Therasse P, Arbuck SG, Eisenhauer EA, Wanders J, Kaplan RS, Rubinstein L, Verweij J, Van Glabbeke M, van Oosterom AT, Christian MC et al (2000) New guidelines to evaluate the response to treatment in solid tumors. European Organization for Research and Treatment of Cancer, National Cancer Institute of the United States, National Cancer Institute of Canada. J Natl Cancer Inst 92:205–216
51. Gianni L, Llado A, Bianchi G, Cortes J, Kellokumpu-Lehtinen P, Cameron D, Miles D, Salvagni S, Wardley A, Goeminne J-C et al (2010) Open-label, Phase II multicenter, randomized study of the efficacy and safety of two dose levels of pertuzumab, a HER2 dimerization inhibitor, in patients with HER2-negative metastatic breast cancer. J Clin Oncol 28: 1131–1137
52. Cortés J, Baselga J, Petrella T, Gelmon K, Fumoleau P, Verma S, Pivot X, Ross G, Szado T, Gianni L (2009) Pertuzumab monotherapy following trastuzumab-based treatment: Activity and tolerability in patients with advanced HER2- positive breast cancer. J Clin Oncol (Meeting Abstracts) 27:46s, abstract 1022
53. ERBITUX® (Cetuximab) Package Insert. ImClone Systems Incorporated and Bristol-Myers Squibb Company (2007)
54. Highlights of prescribing information. Lapatinib (2007)
55. Amler L, Gordon MS, Strauss A, Rabbee N, Derynck MK, Krueger K, Eberhard DA, Matei D, Karlan BY (2006) Identification of predictive markers of clinical activity from a phase II trial of single agent pertuzumab (rhuMab2C4), a HER dimerization inhibitor, in advanced ovarian cancer (OC). J Clin Oncol (Meeting Abstracts) 24:121s, abstract 3001
56. Amler L, Makhija S, Januario T, Matulonis UA, Strauss A, Dizon DS, Sliwkowski MX, Dolezal M, Tong B, Paton V (2008) HER pathway gene expression analysis in a phase II study of pertuzumab + gemcitabine vs. gemcitabine + placebo in patients with platinum-resistant epithelial ovarian cancer. J Clin Oncol (Meeting Abstracts) 26:305s, abstract 5552

Beyond Trastuzumab: Second-Generation Targeted Therapies for HER-2-positive Breast Cancer

Flavio F. Solca, Guenther R. Adolf, Hilary Jones, and Martina M. Uttenreuther-Fischer

Abstract Growth factor receptors of the ErbB family play key roles in transmitting mitogenic and anti-apoptotic signals in epithelial cells. Aberrant activation of these pathways by a variety of mechanisms, including receptor over-expression due to gene amplification and activating mutations in receptors or downstream signal transducers, contributes to tumourigenesis, invasion and tumour angiogenesis. Consequently, these pathways have been the focus of intense drug discovery activities for a number of years, resulting in several approved and development-stage therapeutic agents. These include monoclonal antibodies as well as low-molecular-weight kinase inhibitors. In particular, trastuzumab, a monoclonal antibody specific for the human epidermal growth factor receptor (HER-2) receptor, has provided a major therapeutic advance for patients with HER-2-positive breast cancer, and the drug has often been heralded as the first example of personalised cancer medicine. Unfortunately, as a consequence of the side-effect profile of trastuzumab, a proportion of patients are not eligible for treatment; in addition, primary and acquired resistance mechanisms limit its efficacy. Further research into the mechanisms of resistance suggests that inhibition of additional members of the ErbB family, in particular the epidermal growth factor receptor (EGFR), also known as HER1, may maximise inhibition of the signalling pathways with a resultant improvement in efficacy. This chapter focuses on small-molecule inhibitors of both the HER-2 and EGFR/HER1 kinases that bind to their targets either reversibly (lapatinib, XL647, AEE788) or irreversibly (neratinib, pelitinib, BIBW 2992). The data reviewed here indicate that such inhibitors will be a useful addition to currently available treatment options for women with HER-2-positive breast cancer.

F.F. Solca (✉)
Department of Pharmacology, Boehringer Ingelheim RCV, Dr. Boehringer-Gasse 5-11, 1120 Vienna, Austria
e-mail: flavio.solca@boehringer-ingelheim.com

M. Sibilia et al. (eds.), *Drugs for HER-2-positive Breast Cancer*,
Milestones in Drug Therapy, DOI 10.1007/978-3-0346-0094-1_6,

1 Introduction

1.1 HER-2 and EGFR/HER1 are ErbB Receptor Family Members

Both HER-2 ((also known as *neu* or c-ErbB2) and EGFR/HER1/c-ErbB1) are members of the ErbB family of transmembrane receptor tyrosine kinases, which also includes HER3/c-ErbB3 and HER4/c-ErbB4. These receptors play key roles in transmitting mitogenic and anti-apoptotic signals in epithelial cells (Fig. 1). Aberrant activation of erbB signalling pathways by a variety of mechanisms, including receptor over-expression due to gene amplification and activating mutations in receptors or downstream signal transducers, contributes to tumourigenesis, invasion and tumour angiogenesis. Consequently, these pathways have been in the

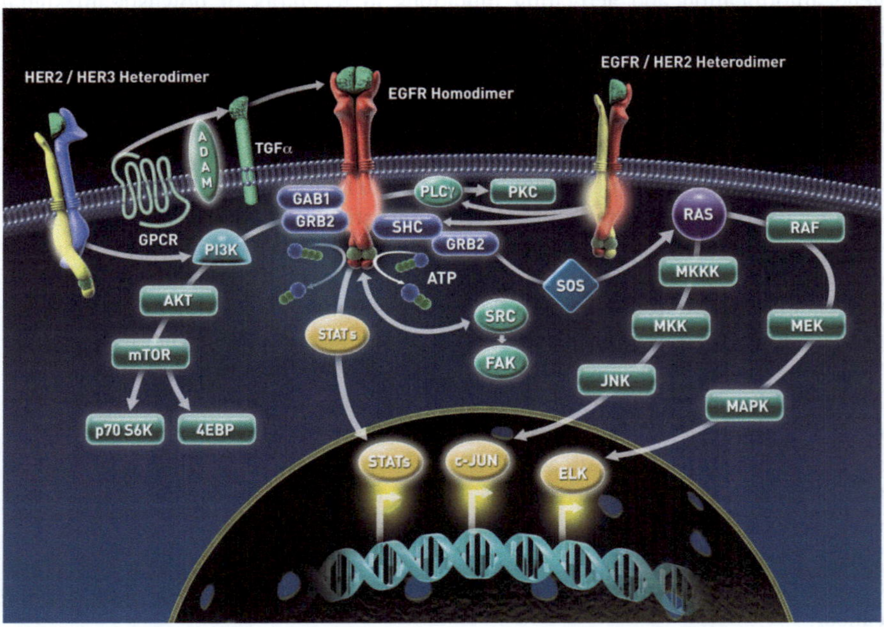

Fig. 1 ErbB receptor signal transduction pathway: Activation of ErbB receptor signalling is mainly dependent on ligand-induced homo- or hetero-dimerisation (both paracrine and autocrine mechanisms described) of ErbB partners and results in transphosphorylation of selected tyrosine residues which act as competent docking sites for intracellular signalling molecules. Ligands (e.g., TGFα) are membrane bound and depend on activation of the ADAM family of metalloproteinases by external stimuli. The main intracellular pathways activated by ErbB dimers are briefly described in the introduction and only schematically outlined here. These comprise the Ras/Raf/MAPK, PI3K/AKT, PLCγ1/PKC, STAT and Par-6 atypical PKC as well as the SRC pathway (for review see [10, 12, 13]). Please note that EGFR can also be referred to as HER1, however for clarity it has only been labelled as EGFR in this figure

focus of intense drug discovery activities for a number of years, resulting in several approved and development-stage therapeutic agents that include monoclonal antibodies as well as low-molecular-weight kinase inhibitors [1–11]. The ErbB proteins consist of three distinct structural domains: an extracellular ligand-binding domain, a transmembrane region and an intracellular tyrosine kinase domain [12]. Upon ligand engagement (at least 13 ligands are known), ErbB members homo- or heterodimerize to form functional units that convey the extracellular signal to the cell interior (Table 1) [13, 14]. Ligand binding induces a conformational change in the extracellular domain that exposes the interaction loop in the CR1 subdomain. This substructure, shared by all ErbB receptors, is responsible for receptor–receptor interaction and allows dimerisation between ErbB family members. HER-2 is unique in that it does not need a ligand for activation as its interaction loop is constitutively exposed [15]. Activation of all other ErbB receptor molecules is mediated by a ligand-dependent mechanism. ErbB3 has no intrinsic tyrosine kinase activity and therefore depends on other ErbB receptor molecules for signal transduction. Ligand-independent activation mainly occurs in disease situations through receptor over-expression or mutations (e.g. EGFRvIII) [12].

Once activated, the dimerized ErbB molecules *trans*-phosphorylate each other on specific C-terminal tyrosine residues. Activation of the intrinsic tyrosine kinase activity requires interaction between the N-lobe of one kinase domain and the C-lobe of the engaged partner [16]. The phosphorylated residues provide docking sites for various proteins including adaptor proteins such as Shc [17, 18], Crk, Grb2 [18], Grb7 and Gab1, kinases such as Src, Chk and phosphatidylinositol 3-kinase (PI3K/AKT), protein tyrosine phosphatases and transcription factors [13, 14, 18]. ErbB receptor dimerisation initiates multiple signal transduction pathways: Ras/Raf/MAPK [17–19], PI3K/AKT [20, 21], PLCγ1/PKC [22], STAT [20, 23] and Par-6 atypical PKC [24]. Activation of these cellular pathways ultimately results in expression of specific target genes that control cell proliferation, resistance to apoptosis, invasion/migration, as well as angiogenesis.

1.2 The Role of HER-2 and EGFR/HER1 in Tumourigenesis

Various mechanisms can lead to aberrant activation of the pathways initiated by HER-2 and EGFR/HER1 including over-expression of ligands for erbB receptors, amplification of receptor genes (e.g., *EGFR/HER1*, *HER-2*), certain mutations in EGFR/HER1 and/or HER-2, transcriptional and translational aberrations, or degradation defects yielding over-expression of EGFR/HER1 and HER-2 proteins [11, 25]. As HER-2 is the preferred dimerisation partner for ErbB receptors, it plays a key role in tumourigenesis in various cancers.

A better understanding of the mechanisms involved in activation of the ErbB receptor pathway and the role of HER-2 in the development of breast cancer led to the development of trastuzumab. Trastuzumab is indicated for treatment of HER-2-positive breast cancer in various settings [26]. However, it has several limitations: It

Table 1 ErbB ligand specificity

ErbB receptors	Ligands													Attributes
	EGF	Hb-EGF	Epiregulin	Epigen	TGF-α	Amphiregulin	Tomoregulin	Betacellulin	Neuregulin				Neuroglycan C	Membrane-bound or soluble
									1	2	3	4		Released by ADAM proteases
c-ErbB1/EGFR/ HER1	x	x	x	x	x	x		x						Activating mutations in NSCLC
c-ErbB2/neu/ HER-2														Over-expression in breast cancer; No ligand binding; Active conformation / preferred dimerisation partner
c-ErbB3/HER3									x	x			x	No intrinsic kinase activity; Multiple PIK3CA docking sites
c-ErbB4/HER4			x	x			x	x	x	x	x	x		Alternative signal transduction mode involving proteolytic processing to target intracellular domain to nucleus

EGF epidermal growth factor, *Hb-EGF* heparin-binding EGF, *NSCLC* non-small-cell lung cancer, *TGF-α* Transforming growth factor-α, *EGFR* epidermal growth factor receptor also described as c-ErbB1, originally discovered as an oncogene (v-ErbB1) encoded by the avian *erythroblastosis* virus. The c-ErbB2 (HER-2/neu), c-ErbB3 (HER3) and c-ErbB4 (HER4) are related receptors discovered later as cellular proto-oncogenes. The human isoforms are also coined HER (*Human Epidermal Growth Factor Receptor Related*) is associated with cardiotoxicity, which makes some patients ineligible and necessitates monitoring in those who receive the drug [26]. It is not effective in all patients with HER-2-positive disease [27]. Furthermore, ErbB receptor pathway blockade by trastuzumab is not complete because it targets only one member in the ErbB receptor dimer and thus development of resistance by HER reprogramming (increased activation of other ErbB family members, such as EGFR/HER1) has been demonstrated as a mechanism for acquired resistance to trastuzumab [28]. Therefore, inhibition of more than one member of the ErbB family is expected to maximise inhibition of mitogenic signalling and could improve efficacy of targeted ErbB inhibitors. Several preclinical studies of the combination of trastuzumab with erlotinib [29] or gefitinib [30–33] in HER-2-positive breast cancer cell lines as well as xenograft models support this concept [34], although some researchers believe that these combinations may not be beneficial in the long run as it is possible that they target only specific subpopulations of cells in the tumour [35]. Reports of the clinical use of these combinations are unfortunately limited. One case report suggests that trastuzumab combined with gefitinib may improve the outcome of metastatic breast cancer [36]. A Phase I trial of erlotinib and trastuzumab provided preliminary evidence of anti-tumour activity [37], whereas a Phase II trial of trastuzumab, gefitinib and docetaxel showed encouraging results [38]. However, it is important to note that not all studies assessing combinations of trastuzumab and gefitinib [39] or erlotinib are positive, thus leaving room for a new generation of ErbB inhibitors that target more than one ErbB family member.

Several other drugs addressing different mechanisms directly or indirectly targeting the ErbB family members are of interest in addressing the limitations of trastuzumab. Pertuzumab, for instance, (a recombinant monoclonal antibody [2C4; Omnitarg] targeting HER-2), is the first representative of a new class of HER-2 antibodies specifically targeting dimerisation and is expected to mask HER-2 to its partners, thereby preventing the formation of active erbB receptor dimers. The heat shock protein 90 (Hsp90), a molecular chaperone involved in the turnover and folding of many proteins, including HER-2, is targeted by several Hsp90 inhibitors currently in development, including tanespimycin, retaspimycin, alvespimycin, SNX-5422, STA-9090, XL888, IPI-493, CNF2024 and AUY922. Histone deacetylases (HDACs) regulate gene transcription by controlling the coiling of chromatin. Dysregulation of HDAC function in cancers may result in oncogene over-expression. HDAC inhibitors currently in development include vorinostat, panobinostat, belinostat, pivanex, romidepsin, valproic acid, ITF2357, MS-275, SB939, MGCD0103, CHR-3996 and PCI-24781. T-DM1 is a novel trastuzumab–drug conjugate that combines the activity of trastuzumab with the targeted delivery of the maytansinoid DM1, a microtubule-disrupting agent, to HER-2-positive cells. T-DM1 is currently in late-stage development for the treatment of breast cancer. Finally, inhibition of both EGFR/HER1 and HER-2 kinase activity, and thus all cancer relevant receptor homo- and heterodimers, is expected to maximise inhibition of mitogenic signalling and to result in improved efficacy [25, 40, 41]. Irreversible binding provides both sustained blockade of receptors, which may improve inhibition of tumour cell proliferation, and activity against receptors that are resistant to first-generation EGFR/HER1 tyrosine kinase inhibitors (TKIs) [25, 40, 41]. Drugs that combine irreversible binding with inhibition of multiple targets offer the greatest opportunity to prevent tumour growth in HER-2-positive breast cancer.

This chapter focuses on small-molecule inhibitors that target both HER-2 and EGFR/HER1, binding either reversibly (lapatinib, XL647, AEE788) or irreversibly (neratinib, pelitinib, BIBW 2992) to the tyrosine kinase domains of these receptors. As most of these compounds are still in development, data are often only available from conference abstracts.

2 Small-Molecule Inhibitors Targeting Both HER-2 and EGFR/HER1

2.1 Lapatinib

Lapatinib (Tyverb®/Tykerb®, GlaxoSmithKline) is a reversible EGFR/HER1 and HER-2 TKI that is indicated, in combination with capecitabine, for treatment of HER-2-over-expressing advanced or metastatic breast cancer after prior therapy with anthracyclines, taxanes and trastuzumab [42]. In molecular kinase assays, lapatinib potently inhibits EGFR/HER1 ($IC_{50} = 11$ nM) and HER-2 ($IC_{50} = 9$ nM) [43] and is also active on the truncated, trastuzumab-resistant form of HER-2 known as p95HER2 [44]. Interestingly, lapatinib is more potent in cells over-expressing HER-2 than in those over-expressing EGFR/HER1 [44]. Thus, the growth-inhibitory effect seems to track more closely with lapatinib's anti-HER-2 activity, despite comparable preclinical inhibitory activity against EGFR/HER1 and HER-2 in kinase assays. Lapatinib's propensity to bind to inactive EGFR/HER1 [45] may explain why this molecule is a less potent inhibitor of constitutively activated EGFR/HER1. Experiments involving treatment of BT-474 human breast cancer xenografts with lapatinib for 77 days showed that lapatinib significantly reduced tumour volume compared with controls, thus supporting clinical trials of lapatinib in breast cancer [44].

Phase II studies demonstrated that lapatinib has activity in HER-2-positive breast cancer both as monotherapy [46–50] and in combination with paclitaxel [51], bevacizumab [52], trastuzumab [53] or tamoxifen [54]. The activity of lapatinib and trastuzumab on biomarker modulation was compared in a neo-adjuvant trial [55]. Complete pathologic responses were observed in 38% of the patients treated upfront with trastuzumab and in 70% of the patients with lapatinib [55]. While cases with low *PTEN* or *PIK3CA* mutations were significantly less likely to show response to trastuzumab, these parameters were not associated with decreased response to lapatinib, providing a possible explanation for the clinical activity of lapatinib in a subset of trastuzumab-resistant patients [55].

In a pivotal Phase III trial, women with HER-2-positive locally advanced or metastatic breast cancer that had progressed following treatment including a taxane, an anthracycline and trastuzumab received capecitabine either alone or with lapatinib. In a planned interim analysis, lapatinib plus capecitabine was superior to capecitabine alone, with improved time to progression (TTP) (8.4 vs. 4.4 months; $p < 0.001$) and fewer disease progression events (49 vs. 72) [5]. In the updated analysis, lapatinib significantly prolonged TTP (6.2 vs. 4.3 months; progression-free survival (PFS) benefit 1.9 months; $p < 0.001$) improved the objective response rate (ORR; 24 vs. 14%; $p = 0.017$) and reduced the number of patients with CNS involvement at first progression (4 vs. 13; $p = 0.045$) [6]. There was a trend to prolonged overall survival (OS) (15.6 vs. 15.3 months; $p = 0.177$), although data were not mature at the time of publication [6].

As paclitaxel (as monotherapy or with carboplatin) is an option for first-line treatment of HER-2-positive metastatic breast cancer [56], a Phase III combination trial was initiated. Paclitaxel plus lapatinib significantly improved TTP (36.4 vs. 25.1 weeks; $p = 0.005$), event-free survival (35.1 vs. 21.9 weeks; $p = 0.004$), ORR (63.3 vs. 37.8%; $p = 0.023$) and clinical benefit rate (69.4 vs. 40.5%; $p = 0.011$) compared with paclitaxel plus placebo in 86 women with HER-2-positive metastatic breast cancer, but at the expense of increased toxicity [7]. Duration of response was increased (32 vs. 24 weeks). Among the 49 patients receiving lapatinib, there were five complete responses (CRs), 26 partial responses (PRs) and nine patients with stable diseases (SDs), compared with 1, 13 and 11, respectively, in the 37 patients not receiving lapatinib. These results are in the same range as previously documented paclitaxel/trastuzumab combinations in the first-line setting, i.e. TTP 6.6–9.0 months and ORR 62–81% [8].

In a third Phase III trial, in untreated postmenopausal metastatic breast cancer, 1,286 women received daily letrozole (2.5 mg) and lapatinib (1,500 mg) or letrozole plus placebo; 219 patients had HER-2-positive disease [8]. In the HER-2-positive population, addition of lapatinib to letrozole increased median PFS (8.2 vs. 3.0 months; $p = 0.019$), ORR (27.9 vs. 14.8%; $p = 0.021$) and clinical benefit rate (47.7 vs. 28.7%; $p = 0.003$). There was no difference in ORR or clinical benefit rate in the HER-2-negative population. At the time of reporting, 41% of patients were still being followed; a possible OS trend was noted in the HER-2-positive population ($p = 0.185$).

Cardiotoxicity is a potential issue for patients treated with trastuzumab. Analysis of safety data from 3,689 subjects treated with lapatinib reported 41 cardiac events among 2,275 breast cancer patients and 19 among 1,038 patients with other tumours [57]. Events were usually asymptomatic, caused reversible decreases in left ventricular ejection fraction and were not related to previous treatment regimen, suggesting that the adverse cardiac effects observed with trastuzumab treatment are drug-related rather than a class effect of HER-2 inhibitors.

2.2 *XL647*

Some TKIs targeting the ErbB receptor pathway, including both XL647 and AEE788, also target vascular endothelial growth factor receptors (VEGFRs).

The VEGFR pathway is involved in angiogenesis, another important target for cancer therapy. XL647 (Exelixis) reversibly binds to EGFR/HER1, HER-2, VEGFR2, VEGFR3 and EphB4 [58]. In in vitro kinase assays, XL647 is a potent inhibitor of EGFR/HER1 and HER-2, as shown by the IC_{50} values of 0.3 and 16 nM, respectively [58]. No clinical data in breast cancer were available at the time of writing; XL647 is currently in Phase I trials in advanced solid tumours.

2.3 AEE788

Similarly, AEE788 (Novartis) targets multiple receptor tyrosine kinases, with potent activity against EGFR/HER1, HER-2 and VEGFR2 [59]. In vitro, it inhibits EGFR/HER1 and HER-2 with IC_{50} values of 2 and 6 nM, respectively. It has anti-proliferative activity against EGFR/HER1- and HER-2-over-expressing cell lines, and inhibits phosphorylation of EGFR/HER1 in A431 cells and HER-2 in BT-474 cells [59]. AEE788 has potent anti-tumour activity in a number of animal models of cancer, including HER-2-positive breast cancer, in which it caused 57% tumour regression at the highest dose [59]. A Phase I trial in advanced tumours has been completed [60] but results are not yet available.

2.4 Neratinib

Neratinib (HKI-272; Wyeth) covalently binds to a conserved cysteine residue in the ATP-binding pocket of EGFR/HER1 and HER-2 [61], and thereby irreversibly inactivates the targeted receptor molecule. Neratinib has been shown to inhibit downstream signal transduction events resulting in G1 arrest and decreased cellular proliferation.

In vitro, neratinib inhibits EGFR/HER1 and HER-2 with IC_{50} values of 59 and 92 nM, respectively [62]. In cellular studies, it is highly active against HER-2-positive breast cancer cell lines, and has limited activity against cell lines that are negative for both HER-2 and EGFR/HER1 [61]. It inhibits ligand-independent HER-2 phosphorylation in BT-474 breast cancer cells at similar doses to those required to inhibit cell proliferation, but EGF-dependent EGFR/HER1 inhibition occurs at a lower dose. Neratinib also attenuates activity of the PI3K/AKT pathway [61]. In xenograft studies, it inhibits the growth of HER-2-dependent tumours.

In a Phase I trial in 72 patients with advanced EGFR/HER1- or HER-2-positive tumours that had failed standard therapy, 7 of 23 evaluable patients with breast cancer had a PR and one had SD [63]. A Phase II study in 136 patients with advanced HER-2-positive breast cancer showed that neratinib is generally well tolerated and has anti-tumour activity in this setting [64]. Response was assessed in patients who had ($n = 61$) or had not ($n = 63$) received prior treatment with trastuzumab, although no information is available on the success or failure of this prior treatment. In trastuzumab-treated and -naïve patients, the ORRs were 26 and 56%; 16-week PFS rates were 60 and 77%, with a median PFS of 23 and 40 weeks, and clinical benefit rates of 36 and 68%, respectively.

Neratinib is currently in Phase III testing with a trial in second-line treatment of HER-2-positive metastatic breast cancer; additional Phase III trials are planned in second and later lines of treatment for metastatic breast cancer, as well as first-line treatment of metastatic breast cancer in combination with a taxane.

2.5 *Pelitinib*

Pelitinib (EKB-569; Wyeth) is a potent irreversible inhibitor of EGFR/HER1 with modest activity against HER-2, as shown by in vitro IC_{50} values of 8 and 378 nM, respectively [65]. Preclinical studies show that pelitinib inhibits growth of EGFR/HER1-dependent A431 cells (IC_{50} 79 nM) and HER-2-dependent SKBR3 cells (IC_{50} 17 nM), as well as growth of A431 tumours in mice after oral dosing at 10–80 mg/kg [65]. However, all further published details on pelitinib involve only EGFR/HER1-driven, not HER-2-driven, models.

There is little information on the use of pelitinib in breast cancer and available data are derived from other tumour types. In the two pelitinib monotherapy Phase I trials reported, pelitinib was well tolerated [66, 67], and no major anti-tumour responses [66] were observed. Pelitinib has been tested in combination with chemotherapy in three Phase I/IIa trials in patients with advanced colorectal cancer with encouraging results [68–70]. It is currently in Phase II trials, but none include breast cancer patients.

2.6 *BIBW 2992*

BIBW 2992 (afatinib; Tomtovok™; Boehringer Ingelheim [*trade name not FDA approved*]) is a potent, irreversible EGFR/HER1 and HER-2 inhibitor suitable for once-daily oral administration [71, 72]. In vitro, it inhibits the intrinsic kinase activity of EGFR/HER1 and HER-2 with lower IC_{50} values (0.5 and 14 nM, respectively) than reported for lapatinib, neratinib and pelitinib [71, 73]. BIBW 2992 induces dephosphorylation of constitutively phosphorylated HER-2 BT-474 breast cancer cells at nanomolar concentrations [74] and inhibits their proliferation in two- and three-dimensional culture systems. In vivo, BIBW 2992 shows potent anti-tumour activity in many human xenograft models known to depend on ErbB signalling [41]. In the trastuzumab-sensitive breast cancer model MDA-MB-453, daily administration of BIBW 2992 at 20 mg/kg induces tumour regression [41].

Interestingly, BIBW 2992 also shows potent anti-tumour activity in a HER-2-positive but trastuzumab-resistant model (SUM 190) known to express large amounts of HER-2 (3^{+} by Herceptest™) and displaying activated EGFR/HER1,

Table 2 In vitro activity of several ErbB inhibitors on SUM 190 cells: the procedure used to determine HER-2 phosphorylation and anchorage independent proliferation of SUM 190 cells was published previously [71]

Compound	HER-2-phosphorylation EC_{50} (nM)	Proliferation (soft agar) EC_{50} (nM)
Trastuzumab	>13,000	>660
Erlotinib	762	226
Lapatinib	68	188
BIBW 2992	30	7

HER-2 human epidermal growth factor receptor 2

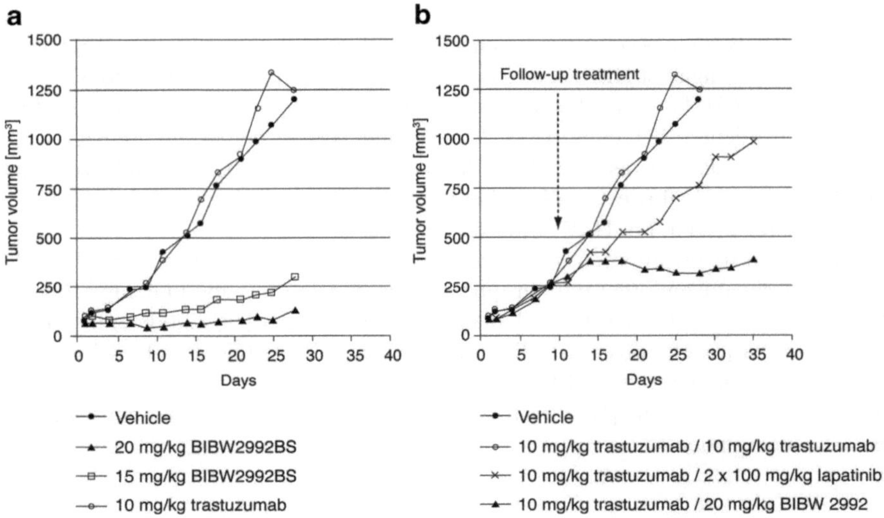

Fig. 2 In vivo activity of trastuzumab, lapatinib and BIBW 2992 in SUM 190 xenografts: (**a**) established tumours (80 mm^3) treated daily with vehicle or BIBW 2992 at indicated doses or bi-weekly (every 3 or 4 days) with trastuzumab; (**b**) all groups were treated with bi-weekly (every 3 or 4 days) trastuzumab until day 11. Follow-up treatments included trastuzumab as described, once-daily treatment with BIBW 2992 or twice-daily lapatinib

HER-2 and HER3 (Table 2 and Fig. 2) [75]. In this model, dephosphorylation of constitutively activated HER-2 was best achieved by BIBW 2992 and lapatinib; erlotinib and trastuzumab only marginally modulated this biomarker, if at all (Table 2). Cellular proliferation was most potently inhibited by BIBW 2992 (median effective concentration 7 nM), suggesting that inhibition of both EGFR/HER1 and HER-2 might be more effective than more selective EGFR/HER1 (erlotinib) or HER-2 inhibition (trastuzumab and lapatinib). In vivo, treatment of mice bearing established SUM 190 tumours (80 mm^3) with trastuzumab corroborated the primary resistance to trastuzumab, whereas treatment with BIBW 2992 suppressed tumour growth in a dose-dependent manner (Fig. 2a). BIBW 2992 was also able to completely suppress the growth of large tumours (350 mm^3), whereas lapatinib-induced tumour growth delay, reflecting in vitro results (Table 2).

While several mechanisms have been described for trastuzumab resistance, "HER reprogramming" involving high levels of EGFR/HER1 ligands activating other ErbB receptors seems to be a possible mechanism for the primary resistance of SUM 190, as high levels of heparin-binding EGF-like growth factor have been measured in this cell line. This mechanism has also been described for secondary (acquired) resistance to trastuzumab in other models (e.g., BT-474 xenografts [28]). Therefore, evaluation of the efficacy of BIBW 2992 in patients with primary or secondary trastuzumab failure seems warranted.

BIBW 2992 monotherapy has been assessed in Phase I dose-escalation studies in patients with advanced solid tumours, including those with breast cancer [76–79]. There are currently only limited efficacy data for BIBW 2992 in breast cancer, but these support the discussed concepts: BIBW 2992 at 50 mg/day in 34 patients with HER-2-positive breast cancer for whom trastuzumab therapy was not effective induced PR in four patients and SD in 14 patients [80].

Further clinical results are available for lung cancer. In Phase I trials, BIBW 2992 treatment resulted in objective response and SD in unselected patients with advanced non-small-cell lung cancer [40, 77, 81]. In preliminary findings from a single-arm Phase II trial of BIBW 2992 in 24 chemotherapy-treated EGFR/HER1 mutation-positive patients, 12 patients had PR and nine had SD [82].

No non-mechanism-related toxicities have been evident with BIBW 2992 in clinical trials to date [40, 76, 77, 83, 84], and dose-limiting toxicities such as diarrhoea and rash are comparable to those of other agents in this class [40].

BIBW 2992 has also been assessed in combination with docetaxel in a Phase I dose-finding study in patients with advanced solid tumours [85]. Of the five patients with breast cancer included in this trial, four derived clinical benefit: one had a CR, two had a PR and one had SD. BIBW 2992 is currently in Phase II trials in HER-2-positive locally advanced and HER-2-positive and -negative metastatic breast cancer.

3 Conclusion

The advent of trastuzumab provided a major advance in the treatment of breast cancer. The limitations of trastuzumab in terms of both efficacy and tolerability are currently being addressed by a wave of low-molecular weight, orally bioavailable inhibitors of ErbB receptor kinases, with encouraging signals of efficacy emerging from ongoing clinical development programs. These NCEs differ in their potency on the EGFR/HER1 and HER-2 kinases and their mode of target binding (reversible or irreversible), with possible impact on efficacy including the development of secondary resistance as well as tolerability. Lapatinib has already demonstrated efficacy in HER-2-positive patients progressing on trastuzumab-containing combination regimens and was approved by the FDA in 2007. The available data thus indicate that the new generation of small-molecule inhibitors are likely to further extend the treatment options for women with HER-2-positive breast cancer.

Acknowledgements This supplement was supported by an unrestricted educational grant from Boehringer Ingelheim GmbH. The author acknowledges the editorial assistance of Ogilvy Healthworld. Boehringer Ingelheim GmbH provided financial support for this assistance.

References

1. Guarneri V, Frassoldati A, Bruzzi P, D'Amico R, Belfiglio M, Molino A, Bertetto O, Cascinu S, Cognetti F, Di Leo A et al (2008) Multicentric, randomized phase III trial of two different adjuvant chemotherapy regimens plus three versus twelve months of trastuzumab in patients with HER-2-positive breast cancer (Short-HER Trial; NCT00629278). Clin Breast Cancer 8:453–456
2. Seidman AD, Berry D, Cirrincione C, Harris L, Muss H, Marcom PK, Gipson G, Burstein H, Lake D, Shapiro CL et al (2008) Randomized phase III trial of weekly compared with every-3-weeks paclitaxel for metastatic breast cancer, with trastuzumab for all HER-2 overexpressors and random assignment to trastuzumab or not in HER-2 nonoverexpressors: final results of Cancer and Leukemia Group B protocol 9840. J Clin Oncol 26:1642–1649
3. Robert N, Leyland-Jones B, Asmar L, Belt R, Ilegbodu D, Loesch D, Raju R, Valentine E, Sayre R, Cobleigh M et al (2006) Randomized phase III study of trastuzumab, paclitaxel, and carboplatin compared with trastuzumab and paclitaxel in women with HER-2-overexpressing metastatic breast cancer. J Clin Oncol 24:2786–2792
4. Buzdar AU, Ibrahim NK, Francis D, Booser DJ, Thomas ES, Theriault RL, Pusztai L, Green MC, Arun BK, Giordano SH et al (2005) Significantly higher pathologic complete remission rate after neoadjuvant therapy with trastuzumab, paclitaxel, and epirubicin chemotherapy: results of a randomized trial in human epidermal growth factor receptor 2-positive operable breast cancer. J Clin Oncol 23:3676–3685
5. Geyer CE, Forster J, Lindquist D, Chan S, Romieu CG, Pienkowski T, Jagiello-Gruszfeld A, Crown J, Chan A, Kaufman B et al (2006) Lapatinib plus capecitabine for HER2-positive advanced breast cancer. N Engl J Med 355:2733–2743
6. Cameron D, Casey M, Press M, Lindquist D, Pienkowski T, Romieu CG, Chan S, Jagiello-Gruszfeld A, Kaufman B, Crown J et al (2008) A phase III randomized comparison of lapatinib plus capecitabine versus capecitabine alone in women with advanced breast cancer that has progressed on trastuzumab: updated efficacy and biomarker analyses. Breast Cancer Res Treat 112:533–543
7. Di Leo A, Gomez HL, Aziz Z, Zvirbule Z, Bines J, Arbushites MC, Guerrera SF, Koehler M, Oliva C, Stein SH et al (2008) Phase III, double-blind, randomized study comparing lapatinib plus paclitaxel with placebo plus paclitaxel as first-line treatment for metastatic breast cancer. J Clin Oncol 26:5544–5552
8. Plosker GL, Keam SJ (2006) Trastuzumab: a review of its use in the management of HER2-positive metastatic and early-stage breast cancer. Drugs 66(4):449–475
9. Johnston S, Pegram M, Press M, Pippen J, Pivot X, Gomez H, Florance A, O'Rourke L, Maltzman J (2009) Lapatinib combined with letrozole vs. letrozole alone for front line postmenopausal hormone receptor positive (HR+) metastatic breast cancer (MBC): first results from the EGF30008 Trial. Cancer Res 69:46
10. Hynes NE, Lane HA (2005) ERBB receptors and cancer: the complexity of targeted inhibitors. Nat Rev Cancer 5:341–354
11. Wieduwilt MJ, Moasser MM (2008) The epidermal growth factor receptor family: biology driving targeted therapeutics. Cell Mol Life Sci 65:1566–84
12. Yarden Y, Sliwkowski MX (2001) Untangling the ErbB signalling network. Nat Rev Mol Cell Biol 2:127–137

13. Olayioye MA, Neve RM, Lane HA, Hynes NE (2000) The ErbB signaling network: receptor heterodimerization in development and cancer. EMBO J 19:3159–3167
14. Scaltriti M, Baselga J (2006) The epidermal growth factor receptor pathway: a model for targeted therapy. Clin Cancer Res 12:5268–5272
15. Garrett TP, McKern NM, Lou M, Elleman TC, Adams TE, Lovrecz GO, Kofler M, Jorissen RN, Nice EC, Burgess AW, Ward CW (2003) The crystal structure of a truncated ErbB2 ectodomain reveals an active conformation, poised to interact with other ErbB receptors. Mol Cell 11:495–505
16. Zhang X, Gureasko J, Shen K, Cole PA, Kuriyan J (2006) An allosteric mechanism for activation of the kinase domain of epidermal growth factor receptor. Cell 125:1137–1149
17. Batzer AG, Rotin D, Urena JM, Skolnik EY, Schlessinger J (1994) Hierarchy of binding sites for Grb2 and Shc on the epidermal growth factor receptor. Mol Cell Biol 14:5192–5201
18. Lowenstein EJ, Daly RJ, Batzer AG, Li W, Margolis B, Lammers R, Ullrich A, Skolnik EY, Bar-Sagi D, Schlessinger J (1992) The SH2 and SH3 domain-containing protein GRB2 links receptor tyrosine kinases to ras signaling. Cell 70:431–442
19. Hallberg B, Rayter SI, Downward J (1994) Interaction of Ras and Raf in intact mammalian cells upon extracellular stimulation. J Biol Chem 269:3913–3916
20. Schulze WX, Deng L, Mann M (2005) Phosphotyrosine interactome of the ErbB-receptor kinase family. Mol Syst Biol 1:E1–E13
21. Mattoon DR, Lamothe B, Lax I, Schlessinger J (2004) The docking protein Gab-1 is the primary mediator of EGF-stimulated activation of the PI-3K/Akt cell survival pathway. BMC Biol 2:24
22. Chattopadhyay A, Vecchi M, Ji Q, Mernaugh R, Carpenter G (1999) The role of individual SH2 domains in mediating association of phospholipase C-g1 with the activated EGF receptor. J Biol Chem 274:26091–26097
23. Bromberg J (2002) Stat proteins and oncogenesis. J Clin Invest 109:1139–1142
24. Aranda V, Haire T, Nolan ME, Calarco JP, Rosenberg AZ, Fawcett JP, Pawson T, Muthuswamy SK (2006) Par6-aPKC uncouples ErbB2 induced disruption of polarized epithelial organization from proliferation control. Nat Cell Biol 8:1235–1245
25. Solca F (2007) Pharmacology and molecular mechanisms of BIBW 2992, a potent irreversible dual EGFR/HER2 kinase inhibitor for cancer therapy. Targ Oncol 132(2):121–132
26. Genentech, Inc. (2008) Herceptin full prescribing information. Available at: http://www.gene.com/gene/products/information/pdf/herceptin-prescribing.pdf. Accessed 3 Dec 2008
27. Krop IE, Winer EP (2008) Ten years of HER2-directed therapy: still questions after all these years. Breast Cancer Res Treat 113:207–209
28. Ritter CA, Perez-Torres M, Rinehart C, Guix M, Dugger T, Engelman JA, Arteaga CL (2007) Human breast cancer cells selected for resistance to trastuzumab in vivo overexpress epidermal growth factor receptor and ErbB ligands and remain dependent on the ErbB receptor network. Clin Cancer Res 13:4909–4919
29. Emlet DR, Brown KA, Kociban DL, Pollice AA, Smith CA, Ong BB, Shackney SE (2007) Response to trastuzumab, erlotinib, and bevacizumab, alone and in combination, is correlated with the level of human epidermal growth factor receptor-2 expression in human breast cancer cell lines. Mol Cancer Ther 6:2664–2674
30. Normanno N, Campiglio M, De LA, Somenzi G, Maiello M, Ciardiello F, Gianni L, Salomon DS, Menard S (2002) Cooperative inhibitory effect of ZD1839 (Iressa) in combination with trastuzumab (Herceptin) on human breast cancer cell growth. Ann Oncol 13:65–72
31. Moulder SL, Yakes FM, Muthuswamy SK, Bianco R, Simpson JF, Arteaga CL (2001) Epidermal growth factor receptor (HER1) tyrosine kinase inhibitor ZD1839 (Iressa) inhibits HER2/*neu* (*ErbB2*)-overexpressing breast cancer cells *in vitro* and *in vivo*. Cancer Res 61:8887–8895
32. Anido J, Matar P, Albanell J, Guzmán M, Rojo F, Arribas J, Averbuch S, Baselga J (2003) ZD1839, a specific epidermal growth factor receptor (EGFR) tyrosine kinase inhibitor, induces the formation of inactive EGFR/HER2 and EGFR/HER3 heterodimers and prevents

heregulin signalling in HER2-overexpressing breast cancer cells. Clin Cancer Res 9: 1274–1283
33. O'Donovan N, Crown J, Clynes M (2006) Dual targeting of EGFR and HER-2 in breast cancer cell lines. J Clin Oncol 24, abstract 13132
34. Narayan M, Wilken JA, Harris LN, Baron AT, Kimbler KD, Maihle NJ (2009) Trastuzumab-induced HER reprogramming in "resistant" breast carcinoma cells. Cancer Res 69:2191–2194
35. Warburton C, Dragowska WH, Gelmon K, Chia S, Yan H, Masin D, Denyssevych T, Wallis AE, Bally MB (2004) Treatment of HER-2/neu overexpressing breast cancer xenograft models with trastuzumab (Herceptin) and gefitinib (ZD1839): drug combination effects on tumor growth, HER-2/neu and epidermal growth factor receptor expression, and viable hypoxic cell fraction. Clin Cancer Res 10:2512–2524
36. Schneeweiss A, Kolay S, Aulmann S, Von Minckwitz G, Torode J, Koehler M, Bastert G (2004) Induction of remission in a patient with metastatic breast cancer refractory to trastuzumab and chemotherapy following treatment with gefitinib ('Iressa', ZD1839). Anticancer Drugs 15:235–238
37. Britten CD, Pegram M, Rosen P, Finn RS, Wax A, Bosserman L, Gordon L, Lin LS, Mass R, Slamon DJ (2004) Targeting ErbB receptor interactions: A phase I trial of trastuzumab and erlotinib in metastatic HER2+ Breast Cancer. J Clin Oncol 22, abstract 3045
38. Somlo G, Koczywas M, Luu T, McNamara M, Bedell V, Slovak ML, Wilczynski S, Morgan R, Russell C, Frankel P (2007) The combination of the HER2 antibody trastuzumab, the EGFR tyrosine kinase inhibitor gefitinib, and docetaxel as first-line therapy in patients with HER2 overexpressing stage IV breast carcinoma. J Clin Oncol 25, abstract 1057
39. Arteaga CL, O'Neill A, Moulder SL, Pins M, Sparano JA, Sledge GW, Davidson NE (2008) A phase I–II study of combined blockade of the ErbB receptor network with trastuzumab and gefitinib in patients with HER2 (ErbB2)-overexpressing metastatic breast cancer. Clin Cancer Res 14:6277–6283
40. Eskens FA, Mom CH, Planting AS, Gietema JA, Amelsberg A, Huisman H, van Doorn L, Burger H, Stopfer P, Verweij J, de Vries EG (2008) A phase I dose escalation study of BIBW 2992, an irreversible dual inhibitor of epidermal growth factor receptor 1 (EGFR) and 2 (HER2) tyrosine kinase in a 2-week on, 2-week off schedule in patients with advanced solid tumours. Br J Cancer 98:80–85
41. Solca F, Baum A, Guth B, Colbatzky F, Blech S, Amelsberg A, Himmelsbach F (2005) BIBW 2992, an irreversible dual EGFR/HER2 receptor tyrosine kinase inhibitor for cancer therapy. Presented at AACR-NCI-EORTC International Conference on Molecular Targets and Cancer Therapeutics (Poster A244)
42. GlaxoSmithKline (2008). Tykerb prescribing information. Available at: http://us.gsk.com/products/assets/us_tykerb.pdf. Accessed 28 Oct 2008
43. Rusnak DW, Alligood KJ, Mullin RJ, Spehar GM, Arenas-Elliott C, Martin AM, Degenhardt Y, Rudolph SK, Haws TF Jr, Hudson-Curtis BL et al (2007) Assessment of epidermal growth factor receptor (EGFR, ErbB1) and HER2 (ErbB2) protein expression levels and response to lapatinib (Tykerb, GW572016) in an expanded panel of human normal and tumour cell lines. Cell Prolif 40:580–594
44. Konecny GE, Pegram MD, Venkatesan N, Venkatesan N, Finn R, Yang G, Rahmeh M, Untch M, Rusnak DW, Spehar G et al (2006) Activity of dual kinase inhibitor lapatinib (GW572016) against HER-2-overexpressing and trastuzumab-treated breast cancer cells. Cancer Res 66:1630–1639
45. Kumar A, Petri ET, Halmos B, Boggon TJ (2008) Structure and clinical relevance of the epidermal growth factor receptor in human cancer. J Clin Oncol 26:1742–1751
46. Lin NU, Carey LA, Liu MC, Younger J, Come SE, Ewend M, Harris GJ, Bullitt E, Van den Abbeele AD, Henson JW et al (2008) Phase II trial of lapatinib for brain metastases in patients with human epidermal growth factor receptor 2-positive breast cancer. J Clin Oncol 26: 1993–1999

47. Burstein HJ, Storniolo AM, Franco S, Forster J, Stein S, Rubin S, Salazar VM, Blackwell KL (2008) A phase II study of lapatinib monotherapy in chemotherapy-refractory HER2-positive and HER2-negative advanced or metastatic breast cancer. Ann Oncol 19:1068–1074
48. Iwata H, Toi M, Fujiwara Y, Ito Y, Fujii H, Nakamura S, Aogi K, Zaks T, Sasaki Y, Takashima S (2006) Phase II clinical study of lapatinib (GW572016) in patients with advanced or metastatic breast cancer. Breast Cancer Res Treat 100, abstract 1091
49. Johnston S, Trudeau M, Kaufman B, Boussen H, Blackwell K, LoRusso P, Lombardi DP, Ben Ahmed S, Citrin DL, DeSilvio ML et al (2008) Phase II study of predictive biomarker profiles for response targeting human epidermal growth factor receptor 2 (HER-2) in advanced inflammatory breast cancer with lapatinib monotherapy. J Clin Oncol 26:1066–1072
50. Gomez HL, Doval DC, Chavez MA, Ang PC, Aziz Z, Nag S, Ng C, Franco SX, Chow LW, Arbushites MC et al (2002) Efficacy and safety of lapatinib as first-line therapy for ErbB2-amplified locally advanced or metastatic breast cancer. J Clin Oncol 26:2999–3005
51. Cristofanilli M, Boussen H, Baselga J, Lluch A, Ben Ayed F, Friaha M, Ben Ahmed S, Hurley J, Johnston S, Kaufman B et al (2006) A phase II combination study of lapatinib and paclitaxel as a neoadjuvant therapy in patients with newly diagnosed inflammatory breast cancer (IBC). Breast Cancer Res Treat 100:S5 [abstract 1]
52. Dickler M, Franco S, Stopeck A, Ma W, Nulsen B, Lyandres J, Melisko M, Lahiri S, Arbushites M, Koehler M, Rugo MS (2008) Final results from a Phase II evaluation of lapatinib (L) and bevacizumab (B) in HER2-overexpressing metastatic breast cancer (MBC). 31st Annual SABCS, December 10–14. Poster 3133
53. Storniolo AM, Magrinat G, Rubin P, Parker B, Rush-Taylor A, Sheidler V, Aranjo S, Shaw C, Eldreth N, Lott G et al (2008) A Phase I, dose escalation study of lapatinib in combination with carboplatin, paclitaxel, with and without trastuzumab in patients with metastatic breast cancer. 31st Annual SABCS, December 10–14. Poster 3121
54. Cardoso F, Koch KM, Awada A, Lokiec F, Brain E, Hayward R, Bogaerts J, Marreaud S, Chung S, Campello V, Fumoleau P (2008) Pharmacokinetics and tolerability of lapatinib administered once daily in combination with tamoxifen. 31st Annual SABCS, December 10–14. Poster 2073
55. Migliaccio I, Gutierrez MC, Wu M-F, Wong H, Pavlick A, Hilsenbeck SG, Horlings HM, Rimawi M, Berns K, Bernards R et al (2008) PI3 kinase activation and response to trastuzumab or lapatinib in HER-2 overexpressing locally advanced breast cancer (LABC). Cancer Res 69(Suppl 2):34
56. National Comprehensive Cancer Network (2009) NCCN Clinical Practice Guidelines in Oncology: Breast Cancer. V.1.2009. Available at: www.nccn.org
57. Perez EA, Koehler M, Byrne J, Preston AJ, Rappold E, Ewer MS (2008) Cardiac safety of lapatinib: pooled analysis of 3689 patients enrolled in clinical trials. Mayo Clin Proc 83: 679–686
58. Gendreau SB, Ventura R, Keast P, Laird AD, Yakes FM, Zhang W, Bentzien F, Cancilla B, Lutman J, Chu F et al (2007) Inhibition of the T790M gatekeeper mutant of the epidermal growth factor receptor by EXEL-7647. Clin Cancer Res 13:3713–3723
59. Traxler P, Allegrini PR, Brandt R, Brueggen J, Cozens R, Fabbro D, Grosios K, Lane HA, McSheehy P, Mestan J et al (2004) AEE788: a dual family epidermal growth factor receptor/ErbB2 and vascular endothelial growth factor receptor tyrosine kinase inhibitor with antitumor and antiangiogenic activity. Cancer Res 64:4931–4941
60. Davis DW, Huang J, Liu W, Xiao L, Thomas A, Mita A, Steward W, Takimoto C, Mietlowski W, Xiong H (2006) Pharmacodynamic analysis of receptor tyrosine kinase (RTK) activity reveals differential target inhibition in skin and tumor in a phase I study of advanced colorectal cancer patients treated with AEE788. J Clin Oncol 24:18S, abstract 3601
61. Rabindran SK, Discafani CM, Rosfjord EC, Baxter M, Floyd MB, Golas J, Hallett WA, Johnson BD, Nilakantan R, Overbeek E et al (2004) Antitumor activity of HKI-272, an orally active, irreversible inhibitor of the HER-2 tyrosine kinase. Cancer Res 64:3958–3965

62. Tsou HR, Overbeek-Klumpers EG, Hallett WA, Reich MF, Floyd MB, Johnson BD, Michalak RS, Nilakantan R, Discafani C, Golas J et al (2005) Optimization of 6, 7-disubstituted-4-(arylamino)quinoline-3-carbonitriles as orally active, irreversible inhibitors of human epidermal growth factor receptor-2 kinase activity. J Med Chem 48:1107–1131
63. Wong KK, Fracasso PM, Bukowski RM, Lynch TJ, Munster PN, Shapiro GI, Jänne PA, Eder JP, Naughton MJ, Ellis MJ et al (2009) A phase I study with neratinib (HKI-272), an irreversible pan ErbB receptor tyrosine kinase inhibitor, in patients with solid tumors. Clin Cancer Res 15:2552–2558
64. Burstein H, Awada A, Badwe R, Dirix L, Tan A, Jacod S, Lustgarten S, Vermette J, Zacharchuk C (2008) Neratinib (HKI-272), an irreversible pan ErbB receptor tyrosine kinase inhibitor: phase 2 results in patients with advanced HER2+ breast cancer. Cancer Res 69:37
65. Wissner A, Mansour TS (2008) The development of HKI-272 and related compounds for the treatment of cancer. Arch Pharm (Weinheim) 341:465–477
66. Erlichman C, Hidalgo M, Boni JP, Martins P, Quinn SE, Zacharchuk C, Amorusi P, Adjei AA, Rowinsky EK (2006) Phase 1 study of EKB-569, an irreversible inhibitor of the epidermal growth factor receptor, in patients with advanced solid tumors. J Clin Oncol 24:2252–2260
67. Morgan JA, Bukowski RM, Xiong H, Clark J, Zacharchuk C, Plazney D, Pelley R, Fuchs C (2003) Preliminary report of a phase 1 study of EKB-569, an irreversible inhibitor of the epidermal growth factor receptor (EGFR), given in combination with gemcitabine to patients with advanced pancreatic cancer. Proc Am Soc Clin Oncol 22, abstract 788
68. Salazar R, Kohne C-H, Tabernero J, Paz-Ares L, Zacharchuk C, Fourneau N (2003) A phase 1/2A open-label study of EKB-569 in combination with CPT-11/5-FU/LV (FOLFIRI) in patients with advanced colorectal cancer. Proc Am Soc Clin Oncol 22, abstract 888
69. Folprecht G, Tabernero J, Köhne CH, Zacharchuk C, Paz-Ares L, Rojo F, Quinn S, Casado E, Salazar R, Abbas R et al (2008) Phase I pharmacokinetic/pharmacodynamics study of EKB-569, an irreversible inhibitor of the epidermal growth factor receptor tyrosine kinase, in combination with irinotecan, 5-fluorouracil, and leucovorin (FOLFIRI) in patients with metastatic colorectal cancer. Clin Cancer Res 14:215–223
70. Tejpar S, Van Cutsem E, Gamelin E, Machover D, Soulie P, Ulusakarya A, Laurent S, Vauthier JM, Quinn S, Zacharchuk C (2004) Phase 1/2a study of EKB-569, an irreversible inhibitor of epidermal growth factor receptor, in combination with 5-fluorouracil, leucovorin, and oxaliplatin (FOLFOX-4) in patients with advanced colorectal cancer (CRC). J Clin Oncol 22, abstract 3579
71. Li D, Ambrogio L, Shimamura T, Kubo S, Takahashi M, Chirieac LR, Padera RF, Shapiro GI, Baum A, Himmelsbach F et al (2008) BIBW2992, an irreversible EGFR/HER2 inhibitor highly effective in preclinical lung cancer models. Oncogene 27:4702–4711
72. Minkovsky N, Berezov A (2008) BIBW-2992, a dual receptor tyrosine kinase inhibitor for the treatment of solid tumors. Curr Opin Investig Drugs 9:1336–1346
73. Spicer J, Calvert H, Vidal L, Azribi F, Perrett R, Shahidi M, Temple G, Futreal A, De Bono J, Plummer R (2007) Activity of BIBW2992, an oral irreversible dual EGFR/HER2 inhibitor, in non-small cell lung cancer (NSCLC) with mutated EGFR. J Thorac Oncol 2:S410
74. Uttenreuther-Fischer M, Solca F, Shahidi M (2007) BIBW 2992, a novel irreversible EGFR/HER2-inhibitor – preclinical results warrant clinical development. Presented at the TraFo, Bergisch Gladbach, Germany, 17–19 May
75. Ignatoski KMW, LaPointe AJ, Radany EH, Ethier SP (1999) erbB-2 overexpression in human mammary epithelial cells confers growth factor independence. Endocrinology 140:3615–3622
76. Shaw H, Plummer R, Vidal L, Perrett R, Pilkington M, Temple G, Fong P, Amelsberg A, Calvert H, de Bono J (2006) A phase I dose escalation study of BIBW 2992, an irreversible dual EGFR/HER2 receptor tyrosine kinase inhibitor, in patients with advanced solid tumours. J Clin Oncol 24, abstract 3027
77. Lewis N, Marshall J, Amelsberg A, Cohen RB, Stopfer P, Hwang J, Malik S (2006) A phase I dose escalation study of BIBW 2992, an irreversible dual EGFR/HER2 receptor tyrosine kinase inhibitor, in a 3 week on 1 week off schedule in patients with advanced solid tumors. J Clin Oncol 24 (18S), abstract 3091

78. Plummer R, Vidal L, Perrett R, Spicer J, Stopfer P, Shahidi M, Temple G, Futreal A, Calvert H, de Bono J (2007) A Phase I and pharmacokinetic (PK) study of BIBW 2992, or oral irreversible dual EGFR/HER2 inhibitor. 14th European Cancer Conference, September 23–27, Barcelona, Spain. Poster 703
79. Awada AH, Dumez H, Wolter P, Hendlisz A, Besse-Hammer T, Piccart M, Uttenreuther-Fischer M, Stopfer P, Taton M, Schöffski P (2009) A phase I dose finding study of the 3-day administration of BIBW 2992, an irreversible dual EGFR/HER-2 inhibitor, in combination with three-weekly docetaxel in patients with advanced solid tumors. J Clin Oncol 27, abstract 3556
80. Hickish T, Wheatley D, Lin N, Carey L, Houston S, Mendelson D, Solca F, Uttenreuther-Fischer M, Jones H, Winer W (2009) Use of BIBW 2992, a novel irreversible EGFR/HER2 tyrosine kinase inhibitor (TKI) to treat patients with HER2-positive metastatic breast cancer after failure of treatment with trastuzumab. J Clin Oncol 27, abstract 1023
81. Plummer R, Vidal L, Li L, Shaw H, Perrett R, Shahidi M, Amelsberg A, Temple G, Calvert H, de Bono J (2006) Phase I study of BIBW 2992, an oral irreversible dual EGFR/HER2 inhibitor, showing activity in tumours with mutated EGFR. Eur J Cancer Suppl 4:174
82. Yang C, Shih J, Chao T, Tsai C, Yu C, Yang P, Streit M, Shahidi M (2008) BIBW 2992 a novel irreversible EGFR/HER2 TKI induces rapid regressions in patients with adenocarcinoma of the lung and activating EGFR mutations: preliminary results of a single-arm Phase II clinical trial. J Clin Oncol 26, abstract 8026
83. Agus DB, Terlizzi E, Stopfer P, Amelsberg A, Gordon MS (2006) A phase I dose escalation study of BIBW 2992, an irreversible dual EGFR/HER2 receptor tyrosine kinase inhibitor, in a continuous schedule in patients with advanced solid tumours. J Clin Oncol 24, abstract 2074
84. Marshall J, Lewis N, Amelsberg A, Briscoe J, Hwang J, Malik S, Cohen R (2005) A phase I dose escalation study of BIBW 2992, an irreversible dual EGFR/HER2 receptor tyrosine kinase inhibitor, in a 3 week on 1 week off schedule in patients with advanced solid tumors. Proceedings, AACR-NCI-EORTC International Conference on Molecular Targets and Cancer Therapeutics 168, abstract B161
85. Schöffski P, Dumez H, Wolter P, Hendlizs A, Besse-Hammer T, Piccart M, Selleslach J, Shahidi M, Taton M, Awada A (2007) A Phase I dose finding study of a 3-day administration of BIBW 2992, an irreversible dual EGFR/HER2 inhibitor, in combination with 3-weekly docetaxel in patients with advanced solid tumors. ACCR-NCI-EORTC October 22-26, San Francisco. Poster B239

Index

M. Sibilia et al. (eds.), *Drugs for HER-2-positive Breast Cancer*, Milestones in Drug Therapy, DOI 10.1007/978-3-0346-0094-1,

MIX
Papier aus verantwortungsvollen Quellen
Paper from responsible sources
FSC® C105338

If you have any concerns about our products,
you can contact us on
ProductSafety@springernature.com

In case Publisher is established outside the EU,
the EU authorized representative is:
Springer Nature Customer Service Center GmbH
Europaplatz 3, 69115 Heidelberg, Germany

Printed by Libri Plureos GmbH
in Hamburg, Germany